Lifechanger

How To Starve Cancer Using Metabolic Strategies & Deep Therapeutic Ketosis

by

Nancy Dennett Ducharme

*This book is dedicated to
Deborah Addario.*

*Keep living your life to the
fullest potential.*

Other Books by Nancy Dennett Ducharme

"*Essential Oils And Cancer: How To Effectively Use The Right Essential Oils To Confuse And Kill Cancer Cells*" - Book One and Book Two (2014)

Coming In 2021: "*The Lifechanger Cookbook: Using The Therapeutic Ketogenic Diet To Kill Cancer Cells And Tumors*"

TABLE OF CONTENTS

FOREWORD

Several years have passed since I wrote my first book, *"Essential Oils and Cancer"* detailing my brother Eric's fight against stage three testicular cancer. I am extremely happy to report that Eric is cancer free and he is doing well. Since those long days of uncertainty and sleepless nights of hoping, praying, and crying for positive results, I have devoted my time searching for solutions to the suffering caused by cancer. It is my sincere wish that others have results like those we were blessed to receive.

Over the years, I have spent thousands of hours communicating with health practitioners and cancer patients alike to compare what works, what does not, and why. I feel that now is the right time to share with you the things that I have learned along the way. What I hope to show you in this book is how to use the power of science to gain control of your healing process. I am not a professional writer nor am I a doctor with my own TV show. I am a woman who will stop at nothing to try and find answers to save the lives of the people I love. That is all.

One of my beloved mentors, Gerry Farr, used to have a saying that had to do with believing in yourself and finding the vision to accomplish one's goals and dreams. He would say, "Nancy, if you stand on the shoulders of giants, even YOU can see farther than the giants." Today, I stand on the shoulders of giants such as biology professor Thomas Seyfried and Dr. Angela Poff. Seyfried and Poff are not just giants in their field, they are true heroes. Without their hard work and dedication to improving the outcome for cancer patients, we would not be on the edge of solving this terrible and heartbreaking disease.

Key Terminology

1. Acetylation - This process determines the amount of energy that proteins use during DNA replication and repair.

2. Acetoacetate – One of the three main ketone bodies created in the liver during ketosis and used for fuel.

3. Apoptosis – Natural self-destruction of a cell.

4. ATP –Adenosine triphosphate. A molecule which provides energy to living cells.

5. Beta-hydroxybutyrate – One of the three main ketone bodies created during ketosis.

6. Chemotherapy – Type of cancer treatment using one or more anti-cancer drug as part of standardized care.

7. Deacetylation – This process prevents genes from being expressed by blocking the accessibility to chromatins.

8. Phenotypes – The characteristics of cells during certain conditions.

9. Mitochondria – Cell organelles that generate most of the energy needed to power the cell's biochemical reaction.

10. Ketosis – A metabolic state where fat becomes the primary source for fueling the body.

11. Ketogenic Diet – A specific dietary plan used to initiate ketosis. The diet is high in fat, moderate in protein, and very low in carbohydrates.

12. Oncogene – A gene which in certain circumstances can turn a cell into a malignant tumor cell.

13. Ketones – Molecules produced by the liver from fatty acids. These molecules provide energy to the body when carbohydrates (glucose) is very low or non-existent.

14. Intermittent Fasting – A way of eating where food consumption is restricted during specific times of the day, or days of the week.

15. Oxidative Phosphorylation - A metabolic pathway in which cells use enzymes to oxidize nutrients and create ATP for energy.

16. Fermentation – A chemical process by which molecules are broken down without the presence of oxygen.

17. Oxidation – A chemical process in which a substance gains oxygen.

18. Oxygenation - A process where oxygen is introduced into the body where it binds to the hemoglobin in red blood cells, or dissolves into the plasma.

19. Hypoxia – An acute absence of oxygen enough to cause damage to cells.

20. Somatic Theory of Gene Mutation – The theory that states that aging is determined by the genes inherited at birth, and that each time a cell divides in the body there is a chance that some of the genes will be copied incorrectly.

21. MCT Oil – Medium chain triglyceride oil. Fatty acids having between 6-12 carbon atoms. They are present in palm kernel oil and coconut oil.

22. HDAC Inhibitors – Histone deacetylase inhibitors. These enzymes remove the acetyl functional groups from histones thus allowing the histones to expand and the chromatins to open and genes to be expressed.

23. Histones – Protein balls that provide the spiral structure of the DNA. When these histones are acetylated, they expand so that the genes can be expressed.

24. Epigenetics - The study of how changes in environment and behavior can affect the alteration of your genes. Examples: Inflammation, Poor Diet, Oxygenation

25. Glutamine – An amino acid that is produced in the body and also found in foods.

26. Glucose – A simple sugar that is a component of many carbohydrates. It is broken down to produce energy for living organisms.

27. Radiotherapy – Also called radiation therapy. In cancer treatment radiotherapy uses high doses of radiation to kill cancer cells and shrink tumors.

28. Hyperbaric Oxygen Therapy – A medical treatment in which breathable oxygen is used in a bariatric pressure chamber to increase levels of O2 in the blood.

29. Phrenic Nerve – A motor/sensory nerve located in the upper torso which regulates the movement of the diaphragm which in turn controls the intake of oxygen.

30. Krebbs Cycle – Also known as the TCA cycle and the citric acid cycle. A chemical reaction used to release energy for fuel from carbohydrates, fats, and proteins.

31. Tumor suppressor gene – A gene that regulates a cell during replication and keeps it from over-replicating and becoming cancerous.

32. NLR3P inflammasome – A protein complex that initiates the release of proinflammatory cytokines. This inflammasome has been linked to diseases such as Alzheimer's and type 2 diabetes.

33. Glioblastoma – A very aggressive form of brain cancer.

CHAPTER ONE

THROUGH YOU

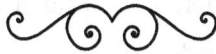

In my life, I have worked with dozens of cancer patients. Finding out that you, or someone close to you, have been diagnosed with cancer can be one of the most devastating moments of your life. It is a moment where even people who have absolute faith in a higher power are shaken to their very core. It is an instance when people start to think about death and their own mortality, perhaps for the first time. It is also a time when people call upon strength for salvation. Some find that strength within themselves and harness its power to take on the greatest battle of their life. Cancer is such a fear for some people that they can only refer to it as 'the C word'. Not being able to say the full word "cancer" feeds into their fear and gives the cancer more power and control than it deserves.

Fearing cancer is normal. According to Cancer Research UK[1], cancer is the most feared disease in the world, named first by about 35% of people in the survey; Alzheimer's disease is second at 25%. The study also reveals that brain cancer is the most feared type of cancer for both men and women. Bowel cancer is second for men, followed by lung cancer and prostate cancer. Breast cancer is second for women, followed by bowel and lung.

In my experience some people cannot process a cancer diagnosis, let alone understand what it means for their future or think about short and long-term treatment plans. They may be too stunned to make rational decisions and remember small details. These are natural reactions but like everything else that happens in our lives, for good or bad, we must manage our emotions. If that time comes, it is my wish that every cancer patient could understand this one core tenet: **Cancer is not something that happens TO you, cancer is something that happens THROUGH you.**

That may sound like a catchy slogan posted on someone's social media feed or a billboard put up for a cancer center at a major hospital complex, but it is not. It's about creating the best possible mindset to begin your battle with cancer. So, what is the difference between cancer happening **TO** you and cancer happening **THROUGH** you? The short answer - **EVERYTHING.**

If you believe that cancer is happening to you, you believe it is something that you do not have any control over. This may leave you helpless to fight against it. When you realize that cancer is happening through you, you can better accept the situation and play an active role in your fight with the disease and the outcome.

When a person feels helpless, they may embrace a "victim mentality." This book has not been written to coddle or encourage you to engage in such a mindset. We have all seen the victim mentality in someone we know. They believe that what has happened to them is a result of the negative actions of others and do not take any responsibility for themselves.

When you are told that you have cancer, you have every right to feel sad, angry, or scared. Taking on a victim mentality, however, is the emotional equivalent of giving up. Patients who give up significantly reduce their chances of beating cancer[2]. Cancer survival rates decrease because the patients are far less likely to take care of themselves and stick to their regiment of treatments, medicine, and doctors' appointments. This book has been written to show you that you can summon up the courage and power inside of yourself to fight.

A few years ago, I helped a woman (let's call her Barb) with her breast cancer battle. Her first mistake was researching her life expectancy online. Doing research is both a blessing and a curse, especially when it comes to health and well-being. From a positive viewpoint, there are many great resources that provide helpful information on how cancer and treatments work and what research is being done to fight different forms of cancer. There are also legions of powerful groups, as well as message boards, on the Internet where people are joining to fight cancer as an army, not as an individual. These groups will do anything they can to educate and empower each other, lift each other up in prayer, and guide each other on their journeys.

If the internet was solely composed of positive, powerful messages, some might view it as the greatest achievement in the history of time. Unfortunately, the Internet is also a place of great misinformation, cruelty, and misunderstandings. You can do 20 minutes of research on any sign or symptom and be convinced that you should go to the hospital immediately because you only have a few weeks left to live! Even information on accredited websites like the American Cancer Association (www.cancer. org) or the Mayo Clinic (www.mayoclinic.org) cannot provide a 100% accurate diagnosis for every single patient. There are always outliers and exceptions, especially in a field like cancer where there is a wide chasm between what we know versus what we do not know.

Barb was so convinced that she had fewer than three years to live that she could not leave her house due to constant tears. Her daily mantra became "Why me? Why did this happen to me?" She became so wracked with fear, that she became a prisoner in her own home and of her own body.

Fortunately, she had a guardian angel looking over her, and I do not mean me. Her daughter's unrelenting compassion and love guided Barb through her darkest hours. Her daughter's out and out refusal to let her mom embrace the victim mentality and give up was instrumental in Barb beating cancer. Her daughter helped guide her to better health and a more positive mindset. Barb was very lucky.

Some cancer patients do not have the support of a family member or friend who is dedicated to making sure they are doing everything possible to beat the disease. Those people have two choices - fight or succumb. This idea is summed up nicely by Tim Robbins's character "Andy" in the movie *The Shawshank Redemption (The Shawshank Redemption, 1994 Castlerock Entertainment)*. Andy wrote a letter to fellow inmate Red (Morgan Freeman) in which he implored him to "get busy living or get busy dying". Both men chose the former - Andy escaped the prison where he had languished for decades convicted of a crime he did not commit, and Red was paroled after more than 40 years on the inside.

The metaphor of being locked in prison is a powerful one for what cancer can feel like. When Andy gets to Shawshank Prison he is scared and shocked and the other inmates bet if he will survive the night. Many men in that facility die a slow death, believing that their lives are over. As they await death, they keep their heads down in resignation of what they believe is their ultimate fate; they feel as though life has nothing left to offer them. For Andy, educated and absolutely convinced that he did not do anything wrong, prison becomes a place to better himself. He helps the prison library get new books, another inmate earns a high school diploma, and even helps one of the guards do his taxes, which leads to him doing all the guards' taxes. After the initial shock of being in prison, he gets busy living life.

People who hear that they have cancer and fall into a victim mentality are the embodiment of the "get busy dying" mindset. For a real-life version of how you can "get busy living", let me tell you the story of Hal Elrod, an inspirational man who has not only defied death once, but multiple times.

Hal was born in 1979 and led a typical life up to age 20 when he took a job as a cutlery salesman, living from paycheck to paycheck. One night in 1999, as he was driving home from a business meeting, he died for the first time. No, that is not a typo. Hal died at age 20 - for six minutes.

Hal was struck head-on by a drunk driver who was going 70 miles per hour. When the first responders arrived at the scene of the accident, the drunk driver was alive with non-threatening injuries. His Ford Mustang had been split in two from the impact of the other car. He was barely alive and as the jaws of life were employed to cut him free from the wreckage, he ceased breathing and his heart stopped. Six minutes later, the paramedics miraculously revived him.

Hal did not actually wake up until he was in the hospital. In addition to his brush with death Hal broke 11 bones. When he became lucid, the doctors told him not to expect much from life. They told him that he would struggle to learn to walk again.

Imagine being told you would live a life of suffering at age 20 with your whole life in front of you. How easy would it be to sink into a deep depression and never return from it? Most people would have understood if he had simply resigned himself to his fate and started preparing for life in a wheelchair requiring constant assistance.

Hal did not do that. Instead, he decided that although his injuries could not be reversed, it did not mean that his future was predetermined. He made peace with what happened to his body because he knew he could not change the outcome of the crash. He could, however, commit to staying positive, embracing whatever came next, and doing everything in his power to live the best life possible. Hal adopted an attitude of gratitude.

Can you imagine laying in a hospital bed barely able to move, constantly hurting, unable to recall what happened, and being grateful for it? To a person outside of the situation, that might seem insane, but Hal counted his blessings. First and foremost, he was not dead. His mind still worked, he had not lost his family, nor they him. The path ahead was not set in stone.

The doctors had not ruled out that he might still make a full recovery. When Hal decided to fight, the word he focused on was "might". His prognosis was that he *might* not walk again. Hal threw himself into rehabilitation and recovery. None of it was easy. His broken bones required multiple surgeries. His muscles complained mightily against the strain of every rehabilitation session and seemed to scream into his ear, *"Why hurt so much trying to take a single step when you could sit in a wheelchair or lay in a bed and let everyone else take care of you?"*

Hal was not a quitter. He pushed himself as hard as he could, day after day, and eventually his body began to heal itself. He finally reached the point where he could stand upright and use his arms and legs again. He made what doctors considered both a full and miraculous recovery. Once Hal was up and about again, he did not want to go back to the life of a cutlery salesman. Clearly, there was a higher purpose and a deeper calling for him. He began by pushing the limits of what his body could do. He started jogging and soon was running marathons, eventually completing an ultra-marathon of 52 miles – all before he turned 30. Less than a decade after doctors told him he probably would never walk again; he ran a double-length marathon.

Hal never let go of his optimism and developed his own system of starting each day. His morning ritual worked so well and allowed him to help so many people that he made it into a book called *"The Miracle Morning"* which became a best-seller upon its release in 2012. In 2019, he released a second book called *"The Miracle Equation"* and later in the same year, started a podcast called *Achieve Your Goal*.

At this point, you might be thinking something along the lines of, "Hey, yeah that's great, but what does that have to do with my cancer diagnosis?" Well, Hal's story is only just beginning.

In October 2016, when Hal was 37 years old, he woke up struggling to breathe. He went to the emergency room where he was poked, prodded, and X-rayed for hours. When a doctor finally came to tell him the findings, it was worse than anyone could have expected. Hal had acute lymphoblastic leukemia

(ALL) - a rare form of cancer that affects just 1.1% of all patients. Even more bizarre is that the disease is most common in children between ages two through five, yet Hal was 37 when he was diagnosed. This form of cancer affects the lymphoid line of blood cells and is characterized by a large number of immature lymphocytes. When Hal got to the emergency room, doctors found his heart, lungs, and kidneys all on the verge of collapsing.

The state of shock was almost overwhelming for Hal. How do you not only survive, but ultimately thrive from what should have been a fatal car crash at age 20, to now being diagnosed with a form of cancer that affects a miniscule amount of the population? Having lived an incredibly healthy lifestyle for the past decade and a half, how could this possibly be happening now?

When he had regained his composure, Hal went to talk to his doctor about exploring holistic healing methods for cancer. The doctor essentially replied that Hal didn't have time and he only had a few weeks to live if he delayed starting chemotherapy.[3] It was true. ALL is an acute leukemia which means it progresses at a very quick pace. Left untreated, it is fatal in a span of weeks or months.

For the second time in his life, Hal was faced with impossibly long odds and decided to accept what happened and do all he could do to make the present and the future better. The doctor said that chemotherapy was absolutely necessary, but Hal had heard good things about holistic healing as well. Instead of giving up one to focus on the other, he put them both to work in aiding his recovery.

As Hal began chemotherapy, he also increased his chances of survival by supporting his immune system with supplements and nutrition. He went even further by continuing to practice the power of positive thinking and being grateful, not bitter, in regard to his circumstances.

Today, Hal is alive and cancer-free. He believes with 100% certainty that supplementing his chemotherapy with holistic healing practices saved his life. Hal's story is a valuable lesson for anyone to learn, not just someone suffering from cancer. Deciding which path to take does not always have to be a "THIS or THAT" scenario. You can embrace both. Hal's story and the lessons learned are a big part of what this book is about. I am going to teach you how holistic, non-toxic approaches will support your body during standard cancer care treatments and can amplify the results. Through a synergistic approach with traditional care we will alter the cancer cells both metabolically and genetically. This is not some fly-by-night solution nor the flavor of the month treatment, but a thrilling set of advancements backed by biology and human trials that have had remarkable, life-changing success.

It took many years for the cancer that you, or your loved one, have been diagnosed with to manifest inside your body. Everything you have done over the course of a lifetime, from the foods you've eaten, to the thoughts you've had, to the emotions you've felt, the habits you've built (both bad and good), and the overall environment that you've been exposed to have led to where you are right at this moment.

This is called epigenetics, and it is the main reason why pharmaceutical companies will never patent a single cure for cancer. Epigenetics looks at how gene activity happens when it is not caused by specific changes in a person's DNA sequence. This is also called gene expression. It is used to describe a process that cannot be inherited. You might share DNA with siblings or parents, but you are not a clone of either one of them. Every human is like a snowflake - we are all so different. How can scientists create a single silver bullet solution that will work for everyone? The answer is that they cannot, but do not be discouraged. This is good news because it gives you the opportunity to self-advocate.

Instead of thinking of your circumstances as life-threatening, I want you to look at this the same way you would look at Type 2 diabetes. If you are not familiar with Type 2 diabetes, it occurs in people whose bodies are not regulating their blood-sugar level properly. They can assist in this regulation by eating a better diet, getting exercise, and taking prescription drugs as prescribed by a doctor. Given proper guidance and personal commitment, Type 2 diabetes is something you can regulate and control for the rest of your life. Cancer is the same. You can use these techniques and treatments to regulate it and take an active role in managing it. You will not fear it.

What you will find is that the way you manage cancer all boils down to what you put into your head, literally. Everything you take in like food, liquid, oxygen, odors, and pollution create a cascade of hormones and other chemicals that affect your 'inner terrain.' The thoughts and emotions that populate your mind will do likewise. Therefore, logic dictates that when you change those contributing factors, your inner terrain will also change.

Key Take-Aways And Action Steps

- Everything you put into your head has the potential to trigger a cascade of positive or negative effects on your "inner terrain". Be aware of things like nutrition, thoughts, odors, and sounds. They can make a big difference.

- Develop an "attitude of gratitude". Start each day by writing in a journal. Make sure you list at least ten things (small and big) you are grateful for each day.

- Surround yourself with positive people. Compile a short list of people you can count on to help you, cheer for you, and support you. This can be friends and family, a counselor, your priest, or members of an online support group.

- Listen to audio books and podcasts. Fill your mind with endless hope and a focus on healing. There are many guided mediations you can use to relax and calm your fears. Remember, you are not alone.

CHAPTER TWO

REVOLUTION

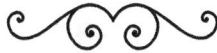

Revolution - *n.* a forcible overthrow of a government or social order, in favor of a new system

Boston, Massachusetts knows a thing or two about revolutions. From the Boston Tea Party of 1773, the city has been the site of great leaps forward and progressive thinking for many years. It has been 250 years since those defining events and now Boston is starting another revolution; this time in the world of oncology. It is the home of the Dana-Farber Cancer Institute, a cancer treatment and research facility that is generally considered one of the top centers for adult cancer care in the country. It has also been ranked the number one facility for cancer care in children by *US News and World Report* multiple times. Dana-Farber treats more than 500,000 patients a year with a staff approaching 5,000[4].

As impressive as Dana-Farber is, a revolutionary approach to attacking cancer is being conducted about four miles west at Boston College. More specifically, it is being done in the Biology Department of Boston College's Morrissey College of Arts and Sciences. That is where Dr. Thomas N. Seyfried, Ph D. goes to work every day to fight cancer in an innovative way. Dr. Seyfried may not ride a horse or own a musket, but he just might be the Paul Revere in the world of cancer research. To fully explain what he is doing and why it matters, we first need to take a step back into the history of cancer research.

The Missing Link

Researching cancer is hardly a new endeavor. Throughout recorded history both the people and the animals who roamed the earth have been plagued by cancer. There is evidence of fossilized bone tumors in Egyptian mummies, along with references to the disease in texts that have survived for millenia far back as 3,000 B.C.[5].

Fast forward to the early 20th century, which was the start of modern medicine. Medicine as we know it today began with scientists who connected the dots between chemistry and biology. During this time, the medical community accepted DNA as the genetic code that gives structure to cells. Furthermore, the idea that viruses, radiation, and chemicals could be cancer-causing agents was beginning to take root. Finally, the foundational theory, which stated that genetic mutations could lead to the development of cancer and that some defective genes were inherited, was initially proposed.

For decades, both the pharmaceutical and medical industries have accepted that cancer is a genetic disease[6]. Within cancer cells are tumor suppressor mutations which *define* cancer as a genetic disease. Tumor suppressor genes are normal genes that tell cells when it is time to die, to repair errors with the DNA code, and to slow down cell division. For a long time, there was no debate, however after reviewing several case studies that involved the cloning of animals with cancer tumor cells, something did not sit right with Dr. Seyfried.

In the 1960s, long before Dolly the sheep had been cloned, science labs were using frogs and mice to slice and dice gene theories. Then, in 1973, a University of Minnesota zoologist named Robert G. McKinnell published a paper called "The Lucke Frog Kidney Tumor and its Herpesvirus"[7]. Four years before McKinnell published his 1973 paper, research and experiments he and his team conducted showed inconsistencies with the genetic cancer theory. They had taken a frog plagued with kidney tumors, removed the nucleus of the cancerous cell in the tumor, then implanted it into the embryo of another frog. The embryo developed naturally into a tadpole as frog embryos have for millions of years, and there was no sign of a malignancy. That was an odd occurrence, but from there things got even more strange for McKinnell and his team of researchers.

The oncogene, the gene transplanted from one frog to the other that can transform a normal cell into a tumor cell, prevented the tadpole from growing into a frog. Instead, it died as a tadpole, with not a single trace of cancer in its system. The mystery for McKinnell and his group was twofold:

- What happened to the oncogene?
- Why did the tadpole not continue to grow into a frog and develop cancer?

A few years later, the work of Dr. Beatrice Mintz proved that it was not just a single species of frog that was seeing these counterintuitive results. An embryologist, Dr. Mintz became a leader in the study of mammalian transgenesis at the Institute for Cancer Research in Philadelphia. Mammalian transgenesis is also known as gene delivery, which introduces foreign RNA or DNA to host cells.

In 1975, Mintz published a study called *"Simian Virus 40 DNA Sequences In DNA of Healthy Adult Mice Derived From Preimplantation Blastocysts Injected With Viral DNA"* in the *Journal of the National Academy of Sciences*.[8] In the study Mintz and a co-researcher cloned a mouse using a malignant cell known as teratocarcinoma. Teratocarcinoma is a malignant germ cell tumor that affects humans and other animals. Male mice of a particular species have a high incidence of testicular teratocarcinomas which makes them useful for experimentation and analysis. Her efforts produced a new, healthy mouse without a trace of cancer. She perfected this technique over eight years using some of the first stem-cell experiments in history[9] This finding, along with McKinnell's earlier in the same decade, went against the widely accepted somatic mutation theory of cancer.

The somatic mutation theory was the driving force of cancer research throughout the 20th century and is defined as an alteration in the DNA of animals that occurs after conception. It can be summarized as the belief that successive DNA mutations in a cell are the reason that cancer develops. The combined research concerning the frogs and mice said otherwise, but scientists and researchers were not about to let the fate of a few rodents and amphibians change the widely accepted theory linking cancer to genetics.

In 2003, researchers at St. Jude's Children's Research Hospital in Memphis, TN released a paper called "*Mouse Embryos Cloned from Brain Tumors*".[10] The team cloned a mouse from a brain tumor cell - the nucleus of what is called a medulloblastoma cell. Medulloblastoma is the most common type of cancerous brain tumor that occurs in children (according to St. Jude's Children's Hospital) The new mouse embryo displayed no evidence of any abnormal cancer characteristics. The phenomenon was not restricted to one species, one type of cancer, one lab, or even one century. These findings supported the previous work of Mintz and McKinnell, but the prevailing school of thought, centered around somatic mutations of genes remained the norm.

Genetics is a ground-breaking field that has given us many breakthroughs and the chance to see who we really are and from where we come. In 1990, the world's largest-ever collaborative biological project known as the Human Genome Project (HGP) began. The project was an international effort to identify and map the structure of DNA in terms of physical makeup and functionality. It was completed in 2003, and two years later, the National Human Genome Research Institute joined forces with the National Cancer Institute to begin a new project - The Cancer Genome Atlas (TCGA).[11]

Given the success of the HGP, the next logical step was to research the genetics of cancer. The research of cancer genetics by TCGA started with a three-year pilot project that focused on characterizing three types of cancer in humans: ovarian, lung, and glioblastoma. A second phase began in 2009, looking at the sequence analysis and genomic characterization of 33 cancer types, including 10 designated as rare. The project was completed in 2014 and the work resulted in a molecular-level map of cancer, something that had never been done. Even though the project was considered a success we are no closer to a singular cure for cancer than we were when the project started.

Finding Answers

While consensus in the scientific community was rooted in the genetic relationship, Dr. Seyfried was convinced that the real answer was elsewhere. After significant research into the causation of cancer, Dr. Seyfried was convinced that cancer did not start growing in the nucleus of a cell. If it did not start there, where did it start?

As is so often the case in science, whether it's Thomas Edison inventing the lightbulb or Alexander Fleming discovering penicillin, there is a fluke or a coincidence that elucidates the moment of truth. For Dr. Seyfried, that moment came in the form of a paper he stumbled upon entitled *"Crosstalk from Non-Cancerous Mitochondria Can Inhibit Tumor Properties of Metastatic Cells by Suppressing Oncogenic Pathways"*[12]. Written by a team from the Department of Molecular and Human Genetics at Baylor College of Medicine in Houston, this 2013 paper refocused Dr. Seyfried's attention on the mitochondria.

If the gene mutations in the nucleus were not the driver of the disease, then the next best place to look would be the mitochondria. To understand what he saw and follow his progression through the next few years, we need to first put ourselves back in high school science class to discuss the parts of a cell and how they function.

The Mighty Mitochondria

What are mitochondria and how do they fit into the equation that Dr. Seyfried and so many others have been pursuing all this time? Mitochondria are organelles that exist in cells and make adenosine triphosphate (ATP) which is the molecule that carries a cell's energy. That means they also play a key role in cellular respiration. ATP is produced via chemical energy found in glucose and similar nutrients. They have their own DNA, their own ribosomes and a double membrane for extra protection. If you remember your biology class worksheets, mitochondria are roughly worm-shaped and exist inside the cell. They are referred to as the powerhouses or energy factories of a cell. The energy-making process uses oxygen brought in by your lungs and pushes out carbon dioxide as a byproduct.

Just like any other part of your body, mitochondria can be damaged by viruses and other foreign invaders. When they are damaged, cellular respiration is affected. If cellular respiration is compromised, the cell's entire purpose and its functionality are in danger of failing and dying. The mitochondria's response is to signal the cell's nucleus for assistance. When that signal is received, the nucleus, acting as the "brain" of the cell, decides whether the mitochondria is worth saving, repairing, or whether it should be designated for apoptosis (cell death). If the nucleus activates oncogenes (cancer genes), the damaged mitochondria not only survive, but grow in number, with the additional cells also having a high propensity for damage. Through mutation, if normal genes promoting cellular growth contain the oncogene mutation, they are predisposed to become cancerous.

When the oncogene mutation occurs, the oncogenes send a signal to the mitochondria to begin backup respiration. The respiration, however, is not through oxygen but through the fermentation of glucose, and in some cases glutamine. So not only are oncogenes resisting the body's natural function to die and be replaced with healthy functioning cells, they are also using the body's own energy to reproduce. In essence - normal cells respire, cancer cells ferment. This process is called the

Warburg Effect, named after Otto Warburg, a professor at the Kaiser Wilhelm Institute for Biology in Berlin. It was there where he began work on the metabolism of tumors and the respiration of cells which culminated in him winning the Nobel Prize in 1931 for Physiology.

How Is Fermentation Different from Respiration?

Cells can create energy by one of two ways: respiration or fermentation. Both methods use carbon in the form of sugar as a substrate (the raw material needed for energy creation). Healthy cells prefer the respiration method, also known as oxidative phosphorylation or aerobic glycolysis to create energy[13]. Respiration is much more efficient than fermentation and creates between 36 to 38 molecules of ATP for every molecule of glucose. Fermentation creates only two molecules of ATP. When the mitochondria are damaged and unable to utilize oxygen, as in the case of cancer, the cells are forced to forgo oxidative phosphorylation in favor of fermentation.

Fermentation is a primitive form of energy production. Millions of years ago, when the Earth's atmosphere did not have enough oxygen to support life, microorganisms used fermentation as their key method of energy production. When most people think of fermentation, they think about the production of certain foods and drinks like wine, beer, and yogurt. Fermentation works the same way within the human body, except that it creates an abnormal amount of waste product from glucose called lactic acid. You may remember the feeling of muscles burning during exercise due to a lack of oxygen; that happens on a cellular level. Lactic acid, in the amounts created by anaerobic glycolysis, cannot be cleared quickly. The result is a very toxic microenvironment that ultimately poisons the surrounding healthy cells, disabling the mitochondria. Then the whole cycle repeats itself.

The big takeaway here is that when oncogenes are triggered, they cause damaged cells to proliferate. First, they deny apoptosis which is the death of an unhealthy cell. Additionally, they are overriding the normal process of cell respiration. An analogy for the role of the oncogenes and the damaged cell is someone who does not pay their electric bill.

Eventually, the power company cuts the connection, and the apartment goes dark. Instead of moving out, however, the person in the apartment makes a few questionable carpentry and wiring decisions and manages to draw power from the unit next door. Now they can watch TV, use the Internet, and make food in the microwave by leaching power from another source. Oncogenes are the microscopic equivalent of the electricity thief. Instead of letting the damaged cell be disconnected from the body, it is kept alive and allowed to multiply using an alternate source of power generation.

The Big Picture

Armed with this critical knowledge of cancer cell metabolism, Dr. Seyfried conducted his own studies and confirmed that normal cells begat normal cells and tumor cells begat tumor cells. When you put the nucleus of a malignant cell into a normal cell there is no proliferation of cancer cells. This is the same conclusion that the scientists who studied frogs and mice came to decades earlier. When you put a healthy nucleus into a cancerous cell, however, the result is even more cancerous growth. Based on this information, Dr. Seyfried pushed back against the idea that cancer is caused solely by genetics. The cancer mutations in the nucleus were only one catalyst for cancer. **The damaged mitochondria are a driving force behind cancer development.**

What does this mean to you, the average person who has received a cancer diagnosis? Or the person who has lost a loved one to cancer and does not want to suffer the same fate or see it happen to someone else they love? **It means quite simply that if we can prevent damage to the mitochondria, we can control cancer itself.**

Key Takeaways and Action Steps

- After years of research Dr. Thomas Seyfried came to believe that damage to the mitochondria – and not the nucleus – is the driving force behind cancer development and growth.

- When healthy mitochondria become damaged, they cannot respire normally. Backup respiration is triggered by the nucleus of the cell in the form of fermentation of glucose (also known as the Warburg Effect). This fermentation of glucose potentiates the development of cancer.

- "Epigenetics" plays a big role in cancer development. Pay attention to chemicals in things like cosmetics, skin creams, shampoos and hair sprays as well as occupational hazards like paint fumes and smoke. These things can cause damage to the mitochondria over a period of time.

CHAPTER THREE

EMERGING EVIDENCE

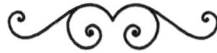

Dr. Seyfried set out to further the theory of cancer as a metabolic disease, not a solely genetic one, particularly as it applied to humans. His efforts ultimately led to the creation of a 2017 paper entitled, *"Press-pulse: A Novel Therapeutic Strategy for the Metabolic Management of Cancer"*. He borrowed the term "press-pulse" from paleontologists who theorized that any mass extinction of living organisms is due to a combination of chronic and acute stressors. For example, a "press" occurrence such as climate change or lack of a food source combined with a "pulse" occurrence like periodic volcanic eruptions, epidemics or a meteor strike could have led to the end of dinosaurs. Next, Seyfried had to figure out the "press-pulse" combinations to weaken cancer tumors.

The obvious choice for the "press" stressor was to cut off all food sources for cancer cells. This was best be done by adopting a diet very low in carbohydrates. Once in the digestive system, carbohydrates easily convert to glucose. The ketogenic diet fit the parameters perfectly - high in fat with moderate amounts of protein and few carbohydrates. The "pulse" stressor turned out to be hyperbaric oxygen therapy, which we will more closely examine in upcoming chapters.

The Press-Pulse Therapeutic Strategy creates a hostile environment for tumors. Through a combination of a calorie-restricted ketogenic diet, pharmaceuticals, and non-toxic therapies (in conjunction with traditional medical treatment) chronic and intermittent acute stress are applied to the tumor. This approach both deprives the tumor cell from nutrients while simultaneously enhancing the positive energy metabolism of the surrounding normal cells. Utilizing Press-Pulse has proven to maximize cancer cell destruction without adversely impacting healthy cell creation and growth. Following are three examples of the impact realized by utilizing this method.

Human Trial #1 - Metabolic Management of Glioblastoma Multiforme Using Standard Therapy Together with a Restricted Ketogenic Diet[14]

In 2010, a 65-year-old woman with glioblastoma multiforme (GBM) was identified for the combination of a standard therapy and a different type of diet. GBMs are the most aggressive type of brain cancer. There is some connection to genetic disorders and previous bouts of radiation therapy, but their causes are unknown. Overall, they represent one or two out of every ten brain tumors that are diagnosed. They are generally found with an MRI scan, a CT scan or through tissue biopsies. There is no known cure for GBMs and once they are found the prognosis is usually fatal. The average survival time after diagnosis is about 12-15 months with treatment. Without treatment, a patient normally lives for an average of three months. Only three to seven percent of people diagnosed with aGBM live longer than five years[15]. The most common form of treatment is surgery to remove as much of the tumor as safely possible followed by chemotherapy and radiation. A medicine called temozolomide is also used, along with steroids, to lower the amount of swelling. Swelling and inflammation in the brain can impact motor skills and neurological function and cause significant pain. However, steroids increase the levels of blood sugar which in turn feed the cancer.[16]

In this case, radiation and temozolomide chemotherapy were recommended while steroid medication was stopped. Additionally, the patient was allowed a water-only therapeutic fasting period and a ketogenic diet (KD) of about 600 calories/day. This diet was supplemented by vitamins and minerals to keep the patient's health intact.

The ketogenic diet forces a person's body to burn stored fat rather than carbohydrates. It has been used to control childhood epilepsy. It also has possible therapeutic uses in many neurological disorders including Lou Gehrig's disease (ALS), Alzheimer's disease, headaches, sleep disorders, and Parkinson's disease[17]. The patient's restricted ketogenic diet was administered at a rate of 4 to 1 (fats to carbs and protein). After two months of treatment, the patient's body weight had dropped by 20% and there was not any brain tumor tissue detected. Biomarkers showed dramatic levels of reduced blood glucose and elevated levels of urinary ketones. This was the first report of confirmed GBM treated with the combination of therapy and the restricted ketogenic diet. The diet was curtailed and ten weeks later the tumor recurred based on MRI evidence.

Human Trial #2: Efficacy of Metabolically Supported Chemotherapy Combined with Ketogenic Diet, Hyperthermia, and Hyperbaric Oxygen Therapy for Stage IV Triple-Negative Breast Cancer[18]

In December of 2015, a 29-year-old woman was diagnosed with Stage IV triple negative invasive ductal carcinoma of the breast. Breast cancer is the most common type of cancer among women, with about 1.7 million new cases per year across the world. It is the leading cause of death by cancer in women and the fifth leading cause overall, leading to roughly 522,000 deaths per year[19]. On a scale of one to three, with three being the most severe type of breast cancer, triple-negative breast cancer usually is graded as a three. Women younger than 50 are more likely to get it, as are African-American and Hispanic women. About one or two out of every ten cases of breast cancer are triple-negative

Incredibly aggressive, this form of cancer tests negative for three common signifiers of breast cancer: estrogen receptors, progesterone receptors, and excess HER2 proteins. As a result, the cancer's growth does not respond to hormonal therapy medicines nor medicines that target HER2 protein receptors. Hormone receptors on the surface of healthy breast cells receive signals from progesterone and estrogen. The hormones attach to the receptors and tell the cells how to grow and function. Breast cancer cells, however, also have hormone receptors that can cause unhealthy functionality. Triple-negative breast cancers do not respond to typical therapies, are more aggressive, and have a worse prognosis than other types of breast cancer. It is more likely to spread beyond the breast and/or recur after treatment.

Around 10 months later, the patient was admitted into the ChemoThermia Oncology Center in Istanbul, Turkey. Doctors there found a tumor in her left breast that measured approximately 3.0 inches by 2.2 inches. Further diagnosis found cancer formations in her upper left abdominal region, her liver, and her axillary lymph nodes.

Her course of action for therapy included standard care, a ketogenic diet, hyperbaric oxygen therapy, and hyperthermia. Hyperthermia is usually given within an hour of radiation therapy and exposes body tissue to temperatures as high as 113 degrees Fahrenheit. As a cancer treatment, hyperthermia can make some cancer cells more sensitive to radiation or harm cancer cells that radiation cannot. It can also damage proteins and structures inside cancer cells or shrink tumors. Hyperbaric oxygen therapy can increase the amount of oxygen in cancer tumors, making them easier to kill with radiation therapy and chemotherapy.

The patient was given a menu of things to eat and not eat. Foods not to eat included bread, pasta, rice, potatoes, sugar, honey, and fruits; she was encouraged to eat vegetables, high-fat dairy, nuts, seeds, meats, and eggs along with following an intermittent fasting schedule. In February 2017, following 12 treatment sessions as well as a KD therapy, the patient showed a total therapeutic response with no lesions present in her left breast, left axilla, liver, or upper left abdomen. Two months later, she underwent a mastectomy of her left breast. The breast tissue showed one lesion but no evidence of live tumor cells. Further tests showed no evidence of cancer.

Human Trials #3: Feasibility, Safety, and Beneficial Effects of MCT Oil-Based Ketogenic Diet for Breast Cancer Treatment: A Randomized Controlled Trial Study

This study took place in 2019 with a group of 60 patients, all of whom were in late-stage breast cancer treatment. There are four stages of breast cancer based on its characteristics such as tumor size and whether the tumor has hormone receptors. The range is from 0 to IV. Stage 0 suggests non-invasive cancers that remain within their original location. Stage IV, also described as late-stage breast cancer, means that invasive cancers have spread outside of the breast to other parts of the body. This stage identification process, known as the TNM system, is overseen by the American Joint Committee on Cancer (AJCC). TNM stands for the size of the cancer tumor and whether or not it has grown into nearby tissue (T), whether or not the cancer is in the lymph nodes (N), and whether or not it has spread to the parts of the body beyond the breast (M). Stage IV is the worst, meaning the cancer has spread into the lymph nodes and other organs including the lungs, skin, bones, liver, or brain. The median survival rate upon reaching Stage IV is three years. The five-year survival rate for Stage IV breast cancer is 22% and the disease kills more than 40,000 people per year in the United States.

The patients in the study were split into two groups of thirty. One group received 12 weeks of a calorie-restricted ketogenic diet along with chemotherapy. The second group received only the chemotherapy. After 30 weeks, 100% of the participants that followed the diet and received chemotherapy were still alive. The group saw significant drops in their fasting blood sugar, BMI, body weight, and percentage of body fat. There were also no side effects regarding their lipid profiles or their liver or kidney markers. Of the group that only received chemotherapy, 60% were alive at the conclusion of the study.The published results concluded that incorporating a calorie-restricted ketogenic diet into a standard care chemotherapy regimen can improve survival while minimizing the side effects caused by chemotherapy.

Key Takeaways and Action Steps

- "Press-Pulse Therapy" is the approach Dr. Seyfried uses to minimize and kill cancer tumors.

- Dr. Seyfried borrowed "press-pulse" from two paleontologists who coined the term after theorizing that a combination of chronic and acute stressors caused the extinction of dinosaurs on Earth.

- The "press" component is the chronic stressor, in this case an anti-cancer diet. The "pulse" component is non-toxic anti-cancer therapy, done periodically such as hyperbaric oxygen therapy.

CHAPTER FOUR

DISMANTLING THE TUMOR USING THE PRESS PULSE APPROACH

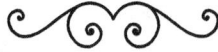

The goal of press-pulse is to attack cancer and, more specifically tumors, from all sides. If you've seen "Return of the Jedi", the last of the original Star Wars films, remember that it ends with a multi-prong battle between the Rebel Alliance and the Empire. The good guys are attacking the Death Star while Luke Skywalker is battling Darth Vader and the Emperor. At the same time, on the planet below, Han Solo, Princess Leia and all those furry Ewoks are using primitive technology to take on the Stormtroopers.

That is a good visual for your battle against cancer using this method. It is about hitting cancer on all sides with various weapons to weaken it in different ways. Some methods are short and focused, some are long and widespread. You put them all together to see what gets the best results and keep blasting your way to victory.

As previously mentioned, it's important to understand that there is no singular treatment, diet, supplement, or therapy that will completely get rid of cancer. To have the best shot at success you must take a synergistic approach that addresses both the metabolic side of cancer origination as well as the genetic side, using every item in your toolbox.

Current standard care regimens include radiation and chemotherapy, both of which are direct, targeted, and periodic. Like a pulse of energy from a sci-fi laser weapon, they attempt to weaken the tumor and the damaged cells. These treatments are heavy hitters. The possibility for bad side effects is always present and therefore they must be used only when necessary and only when the positive outweighs the negative.

The press-pulse method is focused on complementing these treatments by maximizing their efficacy while minimizing their adverse impact. The "press", of the press-pulse method, includes the ketogenic diet and any additional supplements you might take. They are hitting the tumor and the cancerous cells on a daily basis. The constant pressure applied by these two components weakens the tumor and gives it less energy to draw on to promote itself. The "pulse", is intermittent hyperbaric oxygen therapy. Acute and non-toxic, this treatment injects increased levels of oxygen into the bloodstream to weaken the defense mechanisms of the tumor.

The more you know about the process and the research behind it, the easier it will be for you to incorporate it into your treatment and discuss it with your care provider. It also makes it easier for you to stick to the part of the treatment that is entirely in your control – the ketogenic diet. It takes a lot of willpower, a largely new way of thinking, and a commitment to yourself and your body to do the right thing even though it is far from the easy thing.

The Glucose Connection

In the last chapter we learned about German biochemist Otto Warburg and his discovery that cancer tumor cells ferment glucose, even in the presence of oxygen (now known as the Warburg Effect). His Nobel Prize built on the efforts of A. Braunstein from a decade earlier. Braunstein, another German scientist, observed that shortly after diabetic patients were diagnosed with cancer, glucose rapidly disappeared from their urine. His theory was that a tumor overrides normal bodily function and pulls the glucose towards it to fuel growth.[20]

With today's technology, the knowledge that cancer cells consume glucose can be used to see how well treatment is working. Doctors inject a small amount of radioactive glucose into a patient's vein and then use a positron emission tomography (PET) scan to track where the marked glucose is redirected in the body. Because cancer cells are more active and consume more glucose than regular cells they will show up brightly on the scan. This allows doctors to find the location of cancerous cells in the body.

With damage done to mitochondria, cancer cells have no choice but to use the primitive and less efficient method of fermentation. Thankfully, healthy cells have an alternative fuel source option other than glucose. By eliminating the intake of carbohydrates, cancer cells are unable to access glucose while healthy cells can tap into ketone bodies for fuel (known as ketosis). A state of ketosis is achieved when the body uses its own fat stores for energy. The quickest way to enter this state is through fasting.[21]

Fasting is not exactly a new approach when it comes to fighting illnesses. In fact, it was recognized as far back as the 5th century B.C. when it was recommended by the Greek physician Hippocrates. With no new sources of glucose coming in, cancer cells slowly begin to starve and weaken. Fasting produces positive results , there is no doubt about it.

The problem is obvious - the energy you get from eating helps keep you strong and active while undergoing radiation and chemotherapy, however, the addition of fasting to these treatments can make you very weak and sick. It can turn into a case of the solution being as bad as the disease. Fasting is also not sustainable for a lengthy amount of time, particularly if you are trying to live as normal a life as possible between treatments.

A better solution for blocking the fermentation of glucose is to implement the ketogenic diet, a form of nutritional intake that is a key component in the press-pulse therapeutic method.

What is the Ketogenic Diet?

Before we get into the details of the diet, let's talk about the root word. Ketogenic derives from the term ketosis. As mentioned earlier, ketosis is the process that occurs when your body does not have enough carbohydrates to burn for energy. The body then turns to ketones as the alternative source of fuel. To further understand this, we can revisit human history. Before we learned how to farm and domesticate livestock, hunger was a constant, unwelcome companion. When food was available, you ate. Once it was gone, the body relied on the backup energy source of ketone bodies.

The therapeutic ketogenic diet has a multitude of benefits that when combined with other therapies has shown impressive results. The diet is effective in attacking cancer because it mimics the experience of fasting. Instead of starving the whole body, the diet effectively robs the cancer cells of food while supplying the body with a source of sustenance.

Everything humans eat falls into one of three categories: carbohydrates, proteins, or fats. Each is broken down in the digestive system to extract the nutrients vital to human survival. Carbohydrates get broken down into sugars, proteins get broken into amino acids, and fats break down into fatty acids.

However, fats do not break down in the same way. First, they are converted into fatty acids, then into metabolites. Metabolites are the product of the process of metabolism. When fats become metabolites, they are called ketone bodies. There are three kinds of ketones which are created: aceto-acetate, beta hydroxybutyrate, and acetone.

When the fats turn into fatty acid, they do not go through glycolysis - which is the normal method of glucose breakdown - nor do they go through fermentation. Instead they are converted to an enzyme called acetyl coenzyme A. The enzyme enters the mitochondria of individual cells through a series of chemical reactions called the Krebs cycle. Inside the mitochondria of a healthy cell, the enzyme is then converted into ATP which fuels the cells, and thus the rest of the body.

The distinction here is paramount. Cancer cells cannot repeat this process because they lack a particular enzyme (known as the SCOT enzyme) that goes by the tongue-tying name of succinyl Co-A 3-keto-acid CoA transferase.[22] You don't have to remember how to spell it or say it, the most important thing is to remember what it does: convert ketone bodies into fuel. Without this enzyme, fatty acids are as worthless to cancer cells as a bicycle is to a fish.

Since the ketogenic diet is built to rely heavily on fats as the primary energy source, there is far less source material for cancerous cells to use, which in theory should cause them to reduce in size, atrophy and in some cases die altogether.

The Ketogenic diet consists of a high amount of dietary fat, a moderate amount of protein and very few, if any, carbohydrates. The formula calls for around 70% of your daily calories to be composed of fat, 20% of protein and 10% or less of carbohydrates. In using these proportions, the ketogenic diet reduces the amount of insulin being produced by the body.

If you know anything about nutrition, the idea of eating a 70% fat diet probably sets off some warning bells in your head. In the 1980's and 90's we were taught that eating high amounts of fat can lead to all sorts of problems, including cardiovascular disease and high cholesterol. As it turns out, that is not entirely true. It depends on what KIND of fats are consumed. Fats, also called triglycerides, are broken into three different groups – short-chain, medium-chain, and long-chain triglycerides.

Short-chain triglycerides are comprised of less than six carbon chains and they are produced by beneficial intestinal microbes when dietary fiber cannot be digested. They are an important energy source for beneficial bacteria called colonocytes. Next, we have long chain triglycerides which are made up of anywhere between 13-21 carbon atoms. These are dietary oils such as vegetable, canola, and seed oils which can do harm to the cardiovascular system when consumed in large amounts or when heated to high temperatures. Finally, we have the medium-chain triglycerides which have anywhere between 6-12 carbon atoms. The medium-chain triglycerides are further divided up into capric acid, caproic acid, caprylic acid, and lauric acid. All of these can be found in coconut oil.

Medium-chain triglycerides, or MCT's are beneficial because they are metabolized differently by the body. Unlike longer-chain triglycerides, MCT's go directly to the liver where they are converted into ketone bodies. Other benefits of consuming MCT's are lower LDL cholesterol numbers (that's your bad cholesterol), improved HDL (good cholesterol numbers), and an increase in the production of antioxidants.[23]

MCT oils are a main ingredient in many of the recipes in a ketogenic therapeutic diet. The oils aid in delivering the right mixture of nutrients to your body while you undergo cancer treatment. This will give you the best chance of continuing to power your body while diminishing the available energy resources that allow cancer cells to flourish.

Angela Poff, Ph.D., a research associate in the department of Pharmacology and Physiology at the University of South Florida (USF), has been working on ways to use nutritional intervention against cancer, and sees the ketogenic diet as a promising strategy to enhance the results of standard care. In 2018, she appeared on Mike Mutzel's podcast "High Intensity Health"[24] to discuss the subject. She told the audience.

"The ketogenic diet restores anti-tumor immunity. It increases our immune cells ability to attack the cancer and reduces the ability of cancer cells to hide from our immune systems. Our immune systems have the ability to detect and eliminate cancer. Tumors are only a problem when this ability is lost.

We don't always get a remarkable drop in circulating blood glucose. However, with a ketogenic diet you don't get the insulin spikes caused by carbohydrates meals. These spikes potentially drive tumor growth."

For those struggling with cancer, the words "anti-tumor immunity" can make you feel like you're wearing a suit of cancer-proof armor. It's ground-breaking stuff – finding a new weapon against this relentless enemy in our own body. Of course, it's not as easy as eating more fatty food, putting the bread back in the pantry and then watching your tumors shrivel away. Let's take a look at the role insulin plays in the process and what ketones look like when they go head to head with a tumor.

Blocking the Insulin and IGF-1 Pathways

When carbohydrates are significantly reduced in the diet, the amount of insulin in the bloodstream is also reduced. Insulin is one of the most overlooked cancer-promoting factors that can be controlled by diet. When we have a high amount of glucose in the bloodstream, it needs to be shuttled into the cells for energy production. The pancreas receives a signal to start producing insulin - the hormone responsible for storing sugar as energy.

Insulin also has an anti-apoptotic effect on some cancers, meaning it prohibits natural death in cells that have grown out of control. How does this work? The tumors are built to take on insulin in large amounts by having a high number of insulin receptors called IR-A isoforms. The more insulin flowing in a person's body, the more likely cancerous tumors return.[25]

In a study conducted on more than 93,000 women during the 1990s by the Women's Health Initiative,[26] there was significant proof that insulin played a defining role in the recurrence of breast cancer. The study concluded that women with the highest amounts of insulin had more than double the risk of breast cancer returning than women with lower levels of insulin.

Insulin receptors have a counterpart, the Insulin-like Growth Factor Receptors (IGF-1) which become overexpressed in the presence of high numbers of insulin receptors (IR), such as those found on many types of tumors. For example, at least 50% of breast cancer tumors have the BrCa gene. Angelina Jolie had both her breasts removed because she had the BrCa gene which killed her mother. This is the signaling mechanism which triggers the PI-3 kinase cancer pathway, one of the significant pathways leading to rapid tumor growth, proliferation, and survival of cancerous cells. The ketogenic diet can help block these pathways.[27]

Ketones' Effect on Cancer Cells During Standard Treatments

We know that ketone bodies have a positive impact on blocking certain metabolic pathways to cancer, and surprisingly they have also shown great promise in limiting damage done to healthy cells during radiation and chemotherapy.

Radiation and chemotherapy are the real tough parts of cancer treatment. Nobody knows just how tough it is until they go through them. It's sort of like not being able to understand what labor pain is until you deliver for the first time. My brother once explained to me that chemotherapy is like waking up and feeling as if you'd been run over by a truck and were sore in places you had never even realized you could feel pain.

The physical components that are visible from the outside are hair loss, mouth sores, and damage to your skin and nails. However, it goes much deeper. Loss of appetite and nausea are common. Some people are hit hard with constipation, others with diarrhea. Fatigue can flatten you, sapping the energy to do anything. Your concentration and memory can be affected, as can your hearing. Trouble with your muscles and your nerves are not uncommon. The worst part is it might not work at all. There is the possibility that you can endure days and days of chemo treatment - the average cycle is 2-6 weeks - and find that it has had no effect on your cancer. No one should ever have to endure that kind of personal pain and punishment without any results to show for it. Fortunately, new research is showing that the inclusion of the ketogenic diet during these treatments can aid in the shrinking of tumors.

Dr. Colin Champ, MD from the Department of Radiation Oncology at the University of Pittsburgh Cancer Institute ran a study which was published in the Journal of Neuro-oncology in March 2014[28] supporting the efficacy of the ketogenic diet during radiation and chemotherapy treatments. In this retrospective study, 53 cancer patients with glioblastoma multiforme (GBM) were analyzed and their serum glucose levels were tracked between August 2010 and April 2013.

The study compared patients eating a standard diet against those eating a ketogenic diet. Those who were eating the standard diet had an average mean blood glucose level of 122 mg/dl while the ketogenic diet group averaged 84 mg/dl. For comparison's sake, you are considered healthy if your fasting blood sugar level is below 100 mg/dl and your random blood sugar level if below 200 mg/dl. At the end of the study, the data supported the notion that low serum glucose levels during treatment may improve overall outcome.

Ketones as HDAC Inhibitors

Ketones are more than metabolites. Ketones not only have the ability to block cancer metabolically by providing a fuel alternative to glucose, but they can also alter gene expression in the DNA. Chemical compounds called histone deacetylase inhibitors (HDAC inhibitors) are composed of beta-hydroxybutyrate and aceto-acetate. When you look at a strand of DNA, you see the spiraled curled double helix. These are the chromatins. Chromatins keep their shape by wrapping around protein balls called histones. In order for gene expression to happen, the histones have to expand so that the chromatins can be opened, or acetylated. This function is called acetylation because it is caused by the acetyl groups.[29]

In cancer cells the histones and chromatins are stuck in the de-acetylated, or closed position. This is a problem because they need to be opened for the tumor suppressor genes to be expressed. Ketones act as an inhibitor to the de-acetylation malfunction. We see this commonly in the P53 gene mutation, which is a very common occurrence in cancer patients.

Known as the 'guardian of the genome', P53 is a protein that prevents cancer formation and functions as a tumor suppressor in all multicellular vertebrates. P53 repairs DNA so that cancer-causing gene mutations do not get passed onto daughter cells during the replication process. When the P53 oncogene becomes disabled or mutated, it enables and promotes metastasis, angiogenesis, tumor growth, and resistance to cancer drugs. The promise of ketones in the fight against cancer has gained widespread acceptance and major pharmaceutical companies are attempting to replicate HDAC inhibitors to sell as a cancer drug. The good news: you can make your own HDAC inhibitors by getting into a state of therapeutic ketosis.

Article: British Journal of Pharmacology 2008 Feb; 153 (4): 657-668 F. Condorelli, I. Gnemmi(Science article: "B-Hydroxybutyrate: Much More Than A Metabolite" John C. Newman, Eric Verdin, Received August 12, 2014 Division of Geriatrics, University of California, San Francisco)

Exogenous Ketone Supplements and Cancer

If endogenous ketones (naturally created by your liver) act as HDAC inhibitors, what about using exogenous (those taken in pill form) ketone supplements as a part of the diet?

The International Journal of Cancer[30] reported on a study performed at the University of South Florida by Dr. Poff and her associates in which mice were inoculated with the VM-M3 Fluc brain tumor cells. These cancer cells are very aggressive and highly metastatic.

The mice were divided into a control group and a ketone supplemented group. The control group received a standard rodent chow consisting of 60% carbohydrates. The ketone supplemented group ate the same diet, but also received a ketone ester supplement called 1,3-Butanediol (BD) which is a commercially available food additive and hypoglycemic agent. It was combined with saccharin at a 99:1 ratio for taste appeal and then mixed with the food at a ratio of 20% BD mixture to 80% food. The control group received a daily food allotment that was restricted by 40% compared to normal and got their food at precisely 3 p.m. every day. At the end of the study the researchers concluded that the ketones kept the mice alive up to 69% longer than the control group.

Ketones and Inflammation

There is growing evidence that as many as 15% of all cancers diagnosed in the world are attributed to chronic infections. The immune system response causes a cascade effect resulting in the overproduction of reactive oxygen species (ROS). This causes damage and mutations in the nuclear genome, ultimately causing the cell to become cancerous.

Once cancer has taken hold and anaerobic glycolysis is in full effect, the waste product, lactic acid, continues to acidify the microenvironment, creating even more inflammatory damage to otherwise healthy tissue.

The inflammasome, a type of pattern-recognition receptor (PRR), is a vital part of the immune system. Responsible for detecting the presence of many metabolic diseases and auto-immune diseases, the inflammasome targets pathogens and pathogenic microbes and presents antigens to the adaptive immunity system for long-term protection.

First described in detail in 2002, the inflammasome regulates two protective responses: 1) the secretion of cytokines which are pro-inflammatory and 2) the regulation of pyrottosis, a form of cell death. The best characteristic of these is NLRP3, which is named for the protein family it belongs to.

In a 2015 study conducted at the University of South Florida, Dr. Dom D'Agostino and his team discovered that the ketone body known as beta-hydroxybutyrate blocks the

NLRP3 inflammasome.[31] The team found that the NLRP3 inflammasome is associated with the onset and advancement of diseases including immune and auto-inflammatory, multiple sclerosis, inflammatory bowel disease, metabolic disorders, and cryopyrin-associated periodic fever syndrome. The ketone beta-hydroxybutyrate creates a therapeutic effect that reduces the level of inflammation caused by NLRP3.[32]

Ketones May Reduce Chances of Cachexia

Cachexia is a syndrome associated with cancer that causes perpetual muscle loss that cannot be completely reversed with nutritional supplementation. There is not a particular diagnostic criterion for identifying Cachexia, which means it can be difficult to spot until it's in a more advanced stage. It is most commonly found in patients suffering from cancer, as well as chronic kidney disease, obstructive pulmonary disease, and congestive heart failure.

Cachexia strips the body of muscle instead of fat. This occurs because of systemic inflammation that results in changes to the patient's metabolism and the actual composition of their body. About 50% of all cancer patients suffer from it, with the highest occurrence in those suffering from pancreatic cancer or upper gastrointestinal cancer. For those with terminal cancer, it affects nearly four in every five people. For years, the knowledge of cachexia and the way it devastates the body had cancer diet specialists and oncologists encouraging patients to eat as much as they want and whatever they want. High carbohydrates and fats were encouraged. We now know that this is counterproductive to producing ketone bodies.

While it is very understandable why a patient would want to 'bulk up' prior to standard care treatments, it may surprise you to know that the ketone body beta-hydroxybutyrate (BHB) is a muscle-sparing metabolite and can prevent the body from wasting away.[33] BHB was a major component in keeping the species going when man was first learning how to hunt and gather. Imagine people of those times with few structures for protection against the elements, no farming, no domesticated livestock - or anywhere to put them - and no modes of travel outside of their two feet. They were likely nomads who ate an area out of its flora and fauna and then moved on to the next location. Fire was a tool used for cooking but not everyone had access to it, meaning captured meats might have to be eaten raw. BHB allowed people to live without food for a few days at a time when there was no food to be found or if severe weather limited movement. When food was not readily available, the body would kick into ketosis and the ketone bodies would help protect vital organs and muscles from being cannibalized for fuel, in particular the heart and diaphragm muscle tissue.

We've spent a lot of time on the ketogenic diet as a component of the press-pulse therapeutic method of fighting cancer and with good reason. The other parts of treatment are all things that are going to be administered to at a medical facility. While preparation, optimism, and willingness to try things like oxygen therapy, chemotherapy, and others is an integral part of getting through cancer, they are still medical practices that originate outside of you.

Currently, the ketogenic diet requires self-education as it is not widely adopted by doctors or planned by nutritionists. At the end of the day, it will most likely come down to you taking the steps to incorporate it into your lifestyle during treatment. This is not easy, particularly if a high-carb diet has been your staple for a long time, as it is for many. A big key to this diet is having a wide range of fats readily available so that when the craving comes, you have something close at hand to eat or drink. Foods like avocados, nuts, eggs, and fish all have high doses of fat and protein and little to no carbohydrates. If you can grab a handful of nuts instead of a muffin, you'll be on the right track.

Many of us can recall a New Year's resolution to hit the gym four times a week, finally follow that diet, or never eat sweets again only to see it dissolve by Valentine's Day. But this is different. If a doctor tells you to eat a different diet for several weeks in order to lose 15 pounds, you might do it or you may shrug it off when it feels tough. But if a doctor tells you that eating a different diet for several weeks might help take down those tumors and make your other cancer treatments work that much better, that's when it's time to dig deep and think about what matters most. It all depends on your level of commitment.

Hyperbaric Oxygen Treatment

In the Seyfried lab, hyperbaric oxygen therapy (HBOT) is used in conjunction with diet and supplements and standard care to create optimal results. You might have heard of hyperbaric oxygen therapy, maybe you've even used it. Understanding what it is and how it works is essential to the press-pulse approach. Hyperbaric oxygen therapy is a tool used mainly as a medical treatment to stabilize certain conditions such as decompression sickness (the "bends") and carbon monoxide poisoning. The patient is placed in a chamber at 100% oxygen at gradually elevated barometric pressure allowing for maximum O2 absorption in the blood to recalibrate the level of Oxygen in their blood.

A hyperbaric chamber can be a pressurized room or a tube where the air pressure is increased up to three times higher than normal and your lungs gather more oxygen than if you were in a normal environment. This practice is very beneficial to the body because it oxygenates the blood and kills certain harmful bacteria, it calms inflammation, and it also promotes circulation and new growth of blood vessels to feed oxygen and provide nutrients to healthy tissue. In the press-pulse model, HBOT therapy is used to further weaken the tumor prior to chemotherapy or radiation treatments.

A tumor is created under very chaotic conditions. The DNA is mutated, and the tumor vasculature becomes a flawed mass of out-of-control growth. The tumor's blood vessels have holes in them, and there are places within the tumor that have very few or no oxygen pockets. This causes an issue while undergoing radiation therapy.

Radiation works by utilizing oxidative free radicals (ROS), which kill the cells of the tumor, and all surrounding cells, with toxic overload. If there are low levels of oxygen present within the tumor, then there is very little substrate for the therapy to work to create the free radicals needed.

This is where hyperbaric oxygen is beneficial. Doing 90-minute HBOT sessions two or three times per week can help pump oxygen back into areas of hypoxia. This not only increases the odds of successful DNA repair in the healthy tissue in and around the tumor, but it also enhances the impact of radiation and chemotherapy treatments. HBOT also inhibits something called HIF-1 alpha, which stands for hypoxia inducible factor 1, reducing the chances of tumor cell repopulation since the environment becomes inhospitable to anaerobic fermentation of glucose.

HIF-1 prevents apoptosis, or cell death, from happening. It controls pH regulation and metastasis, as well as angiogenesis, by switching on angiogenic factors. HIF-1 encourages the expression of vascular endothelial growth factor (VEGF). Patients with high blood levels of VEGF have a poor prognosis in certain cancers like breast, head and neck, pancreatic, prostate, and renal cancers. Limiting HIF-1 is like cutting the head off the snake when it comes to cancer because it's reduced effectiveness impacts so many parts of the process.

Studies and Citations On HBOT[34]

Combination ketogenic diet, ketone supplementation, and hyperbaric oxygen therapy inhibits metastatic spread, slows tumor growth, and increases survival time in mice with metastatic cancer (123.7)

Angela Poff, Nathan Ward, Thomas Seyfried, and Dominic D'Agostino

Published Online:1 Apr 2014 Abstract Number:123.7

Scholar Commons Citation

Poff, Angela M., "Targeting Cancer Metabolism with Ketosis and Hyperbaric Oxygen" (2014). Graduate Theses and Dissertations. https://scholarcommons.usf.edu/etd/5294

Key Takeaways and Action Steps

- There is no singular diet or therapy, non-toxic or otherwise, that can completely get rid of cancer. A combination of many therapeutic methods can cause a long-lasting positive change within your body.

- For the majority of cancer patients, the therapeutic ketogenic diet is the best anti-cancer diet because it starves the cancer of its number one fuel source and it also creates beneficial metabolites called "ketone bodies".

- Ketone bodies are known as HDAC (histone de-acetylase) inhibitors. These HDAC inhibitors enable tumor-inhibitor gene expression.

- It has been scientifically proven that exogenous ketone supplements can have a positive effect on shrinking tumors.

- Ketone bodies help cancer patients minimize the deadly side effects of cachexia.

- Hyperbaric oxygen therapy (HBOT) pumps oxygen into the hypoxic areas within and around the tumor. This inhibits HIF-1 alpha which block apoptosis.

CHAPTER FIVE

KETOGENIC VS. THERAPEUTIC KETOGENIC

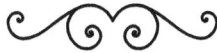

To get the maximum amount of ketone bodies into the bloodstream with the least amount of glucose and insulin, there is a specific guideline that needs to be followed. This is not the traditional ketogenic diet with bacon, eggs, and copious amounts of dairy fat that is used as more of a fad diet by people.

Furthermore, there is a therapeutic benefit to limiting the total daily calories to under 1000. In animal studies involving the ketogenic diet, scientists including Thomas Seyfried noticed that the outcome was more positive when total daily calories were restricted significantly.[35] If that does not sound like very many calories, you are correct, and I won't try to sugarcoat the truth about it. The USDA recommends that we have a maximum intake of 2,000 calories per day for women and 2,500 for men, but that's only a recommendation from a government agency. Neither you nor I are naive enough to believe that most Americans are anywhere close to that figure. According to a report by the Food and Agriculture Organization of the United Nations (FAOSTAT), Americans consume around 3,600 calories per day. Sixty years ago, that number was around 2,880 calories per day. It crossed over the 3,000-calorie mark in the 1970s and passed 3,500 around the turn of the century.[36]

Let's be brutally honest here, more than likely your caloric intake is above the 2,000-calorie count recommended by the USDA. Dropping down to 900 calories is going to be a significant reduction for you. If you are around that 3,600 calorie mark like the average American, it will mean dropping your calorie intake by 75% each day. This will sound terrifying and impossible to you at first, but that does not mean it has to be. Reducing your caloric intake by 75% does not mean the amount of food you eat necessarily drops by 75%, it means that the type of foods you eat are going to change. Some of that will be painful and you will have cravings. That is par for the course for any diet, but as mentioned above, if you educate yourself about nutrition and prepare for those times when your hunger is overwhelming, you can perform a great version of 'mind over matter' and control your stomach and your cravings just like you're learning to control your cancer.

The good news is that this sort of calorie reduction will be temporary, and I will provide you with the step-by-step instructions. Even better news is that you're going to have the chance to learn a lot about nutrition and how different foods break down into different nutrients. This sort of education might be something that has eluded you your entire life as you battle portion size; balance of carbs, fats, and proteins; and getting exercise to keep yourself at a healthy weight. A diagnosis of cancer is a tough price to pay for getting other components of your health under regulation. Those who have used a diagnosis to embrace the rest of their health and make changes across the board will assure you that not only is it possible, but it can be considered a tremendous motivator.

How To Get Into Therapeutic Ketosis

Cutting out the foods that you love and taking a "cold turkey" approach is incredibly difficult. I'm not asking you to do that. Instead, we will reduce your consumption of specific foods over time, easing you into your new cancer-fighting nutrition regimen. In a traditional ketogenic diet, the macronutrients are broken down by percentage. Approximately 75% of daily calories consumed are fats, 15%-20% come from protein, and the remaining 5%-10% come from carbohydrates.

In a therapeutic scenario, the fats consumed daily will equal between 80%-90% of total calories, 5%-10% will be protein, and the remaining <5% will be carbohydrates.

Why the big change and the focus on protein reduction? As we mentioned earlier cancerous tumors prefer glucose, however the amino acid glutamine can also fuel cancer growth. Glucose provides the carbon building blocks for biomass production. Glutamine provides the nitrogen needed for tumor growth and having too much in your bloodstream allows cancerous cells to siphon it off.

We have not talked much about glutamine, but it is a big part of the restrictive makeup of the ketogenic diet. It is found in protein-rich foods including beef, chicken, fish, dairy products, and eggs. Since it gives the nitrogen necessary to spur tumor growth, it must be somewhat restricted. That means that most meats are going to be off the table during the therapeutic phase of the ketogenic diet.[37]

The Glucose/Ketone Index Number

Numbers help us in every facet of dieting. We step on the scale early in the morning to see how much weight we've dropped (or gained, "gulp") since our last weigh-in. We take our pulse rate and our blood pressure to see how much strain we're putting on our heart and lungs to provide oxygenated blood everywhere it needs to be. If we suffer from diabetes, we have the joy of stabbing one of our fingers on a daily basis, or even a few times a day, to check our blood sugar number.

For those using the Ketogenic diet to help aid their cancer treatment, there is the Glucose/Ketone Index. This measurement was devised by Thomas Seyfriend and his team to monitor ketone therapy. Let's break down how this process works step by step. If you've ever done blood tests to get your blood sugar level, a lot of this is going to come naturally to you. But even if you have not, with a little patience you will have it figured out in no time.

There is a scientific formula I'm going to share with you so you can maximize the number of HDAC inhibitors floating around in your body.

The first thing you're going to do is figure out your Glucose/Ketone Index (GKI) number. Before I share the formula to measure your levels, commit to memory that your goal here is for your overall number to be less than three. Why three? Because three is the magic number that tells you that you are in a state of therapeutic ketosis where HDAC inhibitors are being produced in mass quantities to affect the way that tumors are able to take on energy.

The good news is that you can measure your glucose and your ketones at the same time. Using the Keto Mojo monitor (order online at nancyducharme.com) you can get one drop of blood to get readings for both.

A couple of words to the wise about how to prick yourself before you start:

- Don't wash your hands right before you prick your finger. The water and soap will make the blood 'runny' and make it very difficult to collect it properly.
- Don't use the same finger day after day

Once you have accurately recorded both your glucose and ketone numbers, take your glucose number and divide it by 18. If your glucose was 180, you divide by 18 to get 10. If it was 90, you divide by 18 to get 5, and so on. Since most numbers are not divisible by 18, cut it off at the hundredth's decimal for accuracy. For example, if your score is 100, your result when divided by 18 is 5.55.

Next, take that new number and divide it by your keto score to get your Glucose/Ketone index number. Remember, your goal is for that final number be 3.00 or lower to get into the optimal zone for ketosis to happen. When it does, it means your body is burning stored fat for energy. It also means any cancerous cells in your body are getting the silent treatment from carbohydrates, which means a considerable reduction in energy to feed tumor growth. Just to make sure you've got it down, let's run through a couple of examples.

Example 1: Barb takes her fasting blood-sugar and finds it to be 71. Her ketone test reveals a score of 1.7. She takes her blood sugar score and divides 71/18 for a result of 3.94. She divides that by the ketone score of 1.7 and gets a score of 2.32. She is in the optimal zone.

Example 2: Peter takes his fasting blood sugar and finds it to be 133. His ketone test reveals a score of 2.10. Next, he takes his blood sugar score and divides 133/18 for a result of 7.39. He divides that by the ketone score of 2.10 and gets a total score of 3.51. Peter's score is outside the optimal zone. His blood sugar is higher than normal (average range being 65-100 for fasting blood sugar). He must examine what he ate the previous 1-2 days and figure out what carbohydrates he can replace with fats to pull his blood-sugar level down.

There's no shame in struggling with your GKI score and there's a great program called <u>Cronometer</u> that can provide insight into your nutrition and health. It's free to join, and the basic plan is free for life. You can add the food you eat, exercises, other biometric data, and notes about your fitness (a place to store your fasting times and your GKI score).

Based on your current height and weight, Cronometer gives you targets for calories you should be taking in and burning per day, and breaks down the things you eat into energy in terms of calories, protein, fat, and net carbohydrates. As you enter foods you've eaten, it uses a huge database to record the lipids, vitamins, minerals, and proteins that compose each item. It will also break down your carbohydrate count into sugar, fiber, starch, etc. Additional premium features are also available.

When you upgrade, you get access to the app's fasting timer. You can also customize your charts for your specific nutritional needs. This means it can plug in your keto percentages for fat, protein, and carbohydrates and you can track it throughout the day. It allows you the opportunity to do custom biometrics as well and gives you nutrition scores and food suggestions to provide a 360-degree look at your nutrition and health. If you do upgrade, here's how to flip the switch to the ketogenic diet you'll need.

- Go to the dashboard and click "Show full macronutrient breakdown"

- Toggle the button to "Ketogenic" and "Rigorous"

- Change the daily carbohydrates intake to "20 grams of total carbohydrates"

- Change the protein to "0.8 grams of protein per/Kg of lean body mass"

Once set up, you can use this as your daily guideline to monitor your macros. Overall, your DAILY TOTAL calories derived from fat should be between 85%-90%. It's going to be a huge change, but you can do it. This is a pivotal moment in your battle against the cancer trying to take control of your life.

A WORD OF CAUTION: The BRAF V600E Gene Mutation

Before we move further, I need to highlight the BRAF V600E mutation. If you have been diagnosed with any of the following types of cancer: melanoma, colorectal, non-small cell lung cancer, hairy cell leukemia, thyroid, or brain cancer, you must be tested for the presence of the BRAF V600E gene mutation. Some patients with these forms of cancer have this mutation, and if so, must not be on a therapeutic ketogenic diet. There are certain aspects of the diet that will make the disease worse. [38]

What Is The BRAF V600E Mutation And What You Can Do About It

Without exception, all humans are born with the BRAF gene. This gene provides specific instructions for making a protein called B-raf that helps send chemical signals from outside the cell to the nucleus. This signaling pathway is known as the RAS/MAPK pathway, and it controls many cell functions including cell division and growth. BRAF is considered an "oncogene" meaning that it has the potential to cause cancer if it is mutated. When this happens, the chemical signaling from the B-raf protein gets stuck in the "on" position and a cell begins to grow into a tumor.

Roughly 50% of melanoma patients harbor this aggressive oncogene mutation. Approximately 20% of colorectal cancer patients have it as well. About 10% in non-small cell lung carcinoma, 60% of hairy cell leukemia patients, 30% in thyroid gland undifferentiated carcinoma, and less than 10% in gliomas (a type of brain cancer). All in all, there are approximately 30 different BRAF mutations, but the most common is the BRAF V600E which accounts for 90% of all BRAF mutations. Scientifically speaking, BRAF V600E is the result of a single nucleotide mutation resulting in the substitution of glutamic acid for valine at codon 600. A codon is a sequence of three nucleotides which collectively form a unit of genetic code in a DNA or RNA molecule.[39]

The challenge here with the ketogenic diet is that the ketone body produced during ketosis, acetoacetate (AcAc), acts as a fuel for the gene mutation. The ketogenic diet is not a good choice for patients with BRAF V600E. Copper is another nutrient that is required by BRAF V600E, so it's best to stay away from foods high in copper like shellfish, organ meats, and foods with wheat grain during treatment.[40] A good diet would be one low in fat, low in sugar, with a generous number of vegetables and a small amount of meat. You can refer to the BRAF V600E recipes at the end of chapter six for a few examples of recommended ingredients and portions.

Key Takeaways and Action Steps

- There is a difference between a ketogenic and a therapeutic ketogenic diet. The therapeutic diet contains more fat and vegetables, fewer calories, and less meat than the traditional ketogenic diet. The therapeutic diet consists of 1,000 calories or less per day.

- Learn how to calculate your GKI number. GKI stands for Glucose/Ketone Index. If you score a "3" or below, you are in therapeutic ketosis.

- The best way to learn your GKI number is through at-home blood sampling which you can do by ordering a "KetoMojo" monitor on NancyDucharme.com

- If you have the BRAF V600E gene mutation you CANNOT be on the ketogenic diet.

CHAPTER SIX

THERAPEUTIC KETOGENIC RECIPES AND BRAF MUTATION-FRIENDLY RECIPES

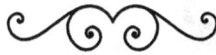

❧❧❧

"Let food be thy medicine, and medicine be thy food." - Hippocrates

Diet plays a huge part in a successful outcome. It is the majority of the "press" portion of the press-pulse strategy. From this point forward, everything you put into your mouth will have an overall effect on your health. Our goal here is to boost the number of ketones floating in your bloodstream, increase the number of beneficial gut microbes, replenish your electrolyte minerals, and cleanse your blood and digestive tract of harmful toxicity.

75

Medicinal Root Tea (*BRAF Friendly*)

The medicinal properties of the roots are used in Chinese medicine to purify the blood. For this tea you will need:

- Lemongrass
- Ginger root
- Galangal root
- Turmeric root

Put a handful of each ingredient into a large pot and fill the pot 3/4 full with water. You may cut the roots into pieces if you'd like. Let it simmer and steep for several hours on low. You may drink this tea hot or cold.

Ketogenic Green Tea

Immune system support is key, the combination of lauric acid from the coconut oil and the acetic acid from the apple cider vinegar is a great combination for supporting the beneficial bacteria living in your gut. Apple cider vinegar also helps support the uptake of minerals in your body while the medium chain triglycerides in the coconut oil primes your liver to start using fat as fuel.

There are four main ingredients in the pumpkin spice mixture – cinnamon, nutmeg , ginger and clove. Cinnamon contains methylhydroxychalcone polymer which mimics insulin and helps to keep your blood sugar levels balanced.

This spice also has cinnamaldehyde which boosts glutathione, a major antioxidant. Nutmeg has macelignan which helps protect the myelin sheath that wraps around the nerves. It's also great for your brain. Next there's gingerol, found in ginger, that helps produce leptin which is a hormone that keeps you feeling satiated. Lastly is clove, which has eugenol that penetrates your cell membranes and keeps the fat in your digestive system from going rancid. You will need:

- 1 or 2 organic green tea bags
- 1 Tbsp organic apple cider vinegar
- 1/4 tsp Himalayan pink salt
- 1 tsp pumpkin spice
- 1 Tbsp organic virgin coconut oil *or* MCT oil
- 1 drop liquid Stevia (optional)

This is a hot water recipe to melt the coconut oil so steep tea bags for 10-15 minutes. After removing the tea bags from your coffee mug, add in the rest of the ingredients and mix thoroughly.

Activated Charcoal Lemon-Limeade (*BRAF Friendly*)

Activated charcoal has been used for centuries to neutralize and flush toxins out of the body. The negative electrical charge of the carbon found in the charcoal naturally pulls harmful positively charged poisons out of the digestive tract. You can use activated charcoal a day or two after having radiation or chemotherapy to help pull harmful remnants out of your system. Just make sure you do not use it for more than two weeks at a stretch. For this drink you will need:

- Juice of 1 large organic lemon, or 2 smaller lemons
- Juice of 2 limes, or 1 Tablespoon Key Lime juice
- 2 Tablespoons Swerve sweetener
- 8-12 oz Cold water
- 1 capsule Activated Charcoal, opened

Put all the ingredients into a large glass, break open the charcoal capsule and drop the contents into the mixture. Stir briskly until the Swerve dissolves. Add ice. Enjoy

Lemon-Lime, Cherry Vanilla, and Orange Soft Drinks *BRAF Friendly*

One of the more difficult items to give up during a ketogenic diet are soft drinks. You can make these drinks mimic the feel and flavor of your favorite carbonated beverages.

Lemon-Lime Soft Drink

- 8-12 oz Sparkling Water
- 1 drop Lemon essential oil
- 1 drop Lime essential oil

- 1-2 tablespoons Swerve sweetener or 5-10 drops of liquid Stevia
- 1 squeeze Organic Lime wedge

Combine all ingredients in a large glass and mix until Swerve is dissolved. Add ice. Enjoy,

Cherry Vanilla Soft Drink

- 8-12 oz Sparkling Water
- 1/4 teaspoon Almond Extract
- 1/4 teaspoon Vanilla Extract
- Tablespoon Swerve sweetener or 5-10 drops of liquid Stevia

Mix all ingredients in a tall glass until the Swerve is dissolved. Add ice and enjoy.

Orange Soft Drink

- 8-12 oz Sparkling Water
- 1-2 drops Orange essential oil
- 1-2 Tablespoons Swerve sweetener or 5-10 drops of liquid Stevia
- 1 squeeze Organic Lemon wedge

Mix all ingredients in a tall glass until Swerve is dissolved. Add ice and enjoy.

Variation: Add 1/4 teaspoon Vanilla Extract for an Orange Cream flavor.

Mineral Broth (*BRAF Friendly*)

This recipe is a fantastic and tasty way to maintain your electrolytes. During fasting you may lose certain minerals like potassium, magnesium and sodium. Sipping this healthy broth can help you replenish them. Please make sure all ingredients are organic and scrubbed clean, and the water is purified. What you'll need:

- 2 Yellow Onions, unpeeled and cut into chunks
- 8 Carrots, unpeeled
- 6 Red Potatoes, unpeeled and cut into chunks
- 6 Celery stalks with greens
- 1 Sweet Potato unpeeled and cut into chunks
- 4 Beets with tops
- 1 strip Kombu
- 4 whole cloves, peeled Garlic
- 2 Bay Leaves
- 6 Peppercorns
- 1 teaspoon Sea Salt

Place all ingredients into a large pot and cover with purified water. Bring to a boil and then turn back the heat to let simmer for 2 hours. Let mixture cool and strain.

Variation: You may add 2 lbs of organic chicken bones to this broth if you wish.

Kimchi (*BRAF Friendly*)

Kimchi is a Korean staple used mainly as a condiment. It takes several days to develop the full effect of fermentation, but kimchi is chock full of beneficial bacteria which helps boost the immune system. It's been proven that maintaining a strong and healthy gut biome during radiation and chemotherapy helps to minimize the harmful side effects. The raw roughage in the kimchi serves as a good prebiotic to feed your gut flora as well, so it gives you double the benefit.

Start off by chopping up two heads of NAPA cabbage into one-inch pieces. Put all the cabbage into a large bowl and sprinkle 2 tablespoons of sea salt onto the cabbage. Massage the salt into the pieces and set aside for one hour.

In a second bowl mix:

- 4 cloves of minced garlic

- 2 teaspoons chopped ginger

- 2 teaspoons sugar

- 2 tablespoons fish sauce

- 2 tablespoons Korean red pepper powder (no substitutions)

- 2 tablespoons sea salt

After one hour, drain the cabbage and rinse off the salt with cold water. Then place the cabbage into the large bowl with the rest of the ingredients. Mix well.

Place the cabbage into a large glass container with air-tight lid. Make sure you fill the container all the way to the top. Press down the cabbage with your hand until the cabbage is submerged in its own juices. Let sit at room temperature for at least 24 hours. The longer you leave it out at room temperature before refrigerating , the more potent your kimchi will be. I usually leave mine out at room temp for five days.

Tossed Salad with Spicy Asian Avocado Dressing

Recipe courtesy of Sharon Merriman, Registered Wellness Practitioner

Ingredients

- 1/2 Ripe Avocado
- 1/2-1 tsp Wasabi Paste
- 1 tsp Coconut Aminos
- 1/4 tsp Fish Sauce
- 1/2 Tbs Toasted Sesame Oil
- 1 clove Garlic
- 1 tsp Raw Ginger Root grated
- 1 Tbs Rice Vinegar

- 1-2 cup Lettuce
- 1/4 cup Napa Cabbage
- 1/4 small Onion
- 1 small Tomato
- 1/4 cup chopped Cucumber
- 4 Kalamata Olives, sliced
- 1 wedge Lime

In a large bowl, mash avocado with wasabi paste, coconut aminos, fish sauce, sesame oil, and rice vinegar. Add all other ingredients except for lime juice. Toss well. Squeeze lime over the mixture, then toss again. Serve.

New England Fish Chowder

I was born and raised on the Seacoast of New Hampshire. New England fish chowder is a definite comfort food for me and it's a dish I enjoy year-round. This is my own recipe, modified for a ketogenic diet. I use wild caught haddock in my recipe, but you can use any kind of firm white fish - cod, grouper, etc.

Ingredients:

- 3 Tablespoons Grass-fed Butter
- 1 clove Garlic, peeled and pounded
- 2 cups Yellow Onion, peeled and diced
- 2 1/2 cups Clam Juice, or Fish Stock

- 2 1/2 cups Heavy Cream
- 2 1/2 lbs. Wild-caught Haddock, or white fish, skinned, boned and cut into chunks
- 1 teaspoon Sea Salt
- 1 teaspoon Old Bay seasoning
- 2 large sprigs Fresh Thyme
- 1 Bay Leaf
- 1/2 teaspoon White Pepper

In a large pot, on medium heat, melt the butter. Add the garlic clove and the onion. Saute' until the onion is transparent. Add the stock, cream, and all seasonings. Maintain a simmer and add the fish. Cook on medium heat until the fish is cooked through. About 40 minutes. Makes six servings.

Summer Vegetable Soup (*BRAF Friendly*)

- 3 large carrots, medium chopped
- 3 medium celery stalks, medium chopped
- 3 cups bell peppers, medium chopped
- 2 medium zucchini, medium chopped
- 2 medium summer squash chopped
- 1 small bag baby spinach leaves
- 1 medium onion, finely chopped
- 6 cups vegetable stock, or mineral broth (see recipe)

- 28 oz can diced tomatoes

- 2 bay leaves

- 1 tsp smoked paprika

- 1 tsp dried oregano

- 1 tsp garlic powder

- 3/4 tsp salt

- Ground black pepper, to taste

- 1 medium garlic clove, minced

- 2 Tablespoons Grass-fed Butter

In a large pot over medium heat, melt the butter and add the minced garlic clove. Add the onion, celery stalks, bell pepper, and cook thoroughly. Add the rest of the ingredients and seasonings and let simmer on medium heat until all the vegetables are cooked through. You may garnish this with Parmesan cheese if you wish. Drizzle with MCT oil for added fat. Makes eight servings.

Vanilla Key Lime Mousse

For when you have a craving for something sweet and tangy. You can adjust the ingredients to suit your own taste. Regardless, this recipe is chock full of MCT oils.

In a blender:

- 3 Avocados, ripened

- 1/4 cup Organic Virgin Coconut Oil

- 2 Tablespoons Key Lime juice, or juice of 3-4 Organic Limes

- 1 teaspoon Organic Lime zest

- 1 teaspoon Vanilla Extract

- 2 Tablespoons Swerve sweetener

Blend until silky smooth. You can adjust the sweetness and tartness however you like. Serves 3

Spinach Roasted Red Pepper and Broccoli Bake (*BRAF Friendly*)

- Oil

- 4 Roasted red peppers, sliced from jar

- 1 cup Baby spinach, raw

- 2 ½ cups Broccoli, blanched and chopped into bite-sized pieces

- 1 small yellow Onion, diced

- 8 Eggs

- ¼ cup Milk

- ½ Parmesan Cheese, grated

- Salt and Pepper to taste

Heat 1 tablespoon oil in a large overproof frying pan. Add onion, peppers, spinach, and broccoli. Stir on medium heat for three minutes. In a separate bowl, whisk eggs and milk. Season with salt and pepper if desired. Pour mixture onto the vegetables and pull the edges of the mixture with a wooden spoon until the eggs start to set.

Heat oven to "broil". Sprinkle frittata with cheese and set under the broiler for 5 minutes.

Serve with a large garden salad.

BRAF-Friendly Breakfast Bowl

- ½ cup diced cooked sweet potato
- 1 cup baby spinach leaves
- ½ cup chopped zucchini
- 1 egg
- pinch of cumin
- pinch of garlic powder
- pinch onion powder
- 2 tbsp coconut oil
- salt and pepper
- salsa

Over medium heat cook the zucchini in the oil until tender then add the spinach. Season with salt and pepper.

when spinach is wilted, remove from the heat. Transfer to your bowl.

Next, add more oil to the pan and warm up the sweet potato.. mash them with a fork and mix in the salt, pepper, and spices. Transfer to the bowl.

Quickly rinse your pan and return to the stove with a little coconut oil. Crack an egg into the pan over medium heat. I always season my eggs with a bit of salt and pepper while they cook, and take it off the heat once the white is set but the yolk is still running.

Spoon a little bit of salsa over the veggie bowl and then gently place your egg on top.

Break the yolk, mix, and enjoy!

Cauliflower Oatmeal

(Cauliflower oatmeal? Yes, don't knock it)

- 1 cup cauliflower rice (Pulse cauliflower in a food processor until it resembles rice)
- 1/2 cup unsweetened almond milk
- 1/2 teaspoon cinnamon
- 1/2 teaspoon Swerve
- 1/2 teaspoon vanilla
- 1/2 tablespoon peanut butter (optional)
- 1 tablespoon psyllium husk

Place the first five ingredients into a sauce pan. Once the pot is boiling turn the heat back to medium, stirring vigorously until the cauliflower is tender.

Once the cauliflower is done, transfer to a bowl and add the peanut butter and psyllium husks.

Vegetable Frittata

- vegetable cooking spray (nonstick)
- 1 onion (medium)
- 1 red bell pepper (medium)
- 1 green bell pepper (medium)
- 1 zucchini (medium)
- 1 teaspoon sugar
- 3/4 teaspoon salt
- 1/4 teaspoon coarsely ground black pepper
- 1/4 cup water
- 4 tablespoons fresh basil (finely chopped)
- 6 large egg whites
- 2 large eggs
- 2 ounces feta cheese

Preheat the oven to 375 degrees.

Grease a non-stick skillet with cooking spray and place over medium-high heat. Add the onion and cook, stirring frequently, until soft and lightly browned.

Add the bell peppers, zucchini, sugar, salt, and pepper. Cook, stirring frequently, until the vegetables are crisp-tender.

Add the water to the skillet and bring to a boil. Reduce the heat to a simmer, cover the skillet, and let cook for 10 minutes. Remove the pan from the heat and stir in half of the basil.

In a bowl, whisk together the egg whites, eggs, half of the feta, and the remaining basil.

Grease an oven-safe skillet with cooking spray. Add the egg mixture and cook over medium-high heat for 2 minutes or until the eggs begin to set.

Remove the pan from the heat. Top the egg with the cooked vegetables and sprinkle with the remaining feta cheese.

Place the skillet in the oven and cook until the cheese has melted and the frittata is set.

Remove from the oven and cut into wedges to serve.

Tinola Soup

Tinola is a wonderful and comforting Filipino favorite

- 3 tablespoons coconut oil
- ½ cup chopped yellow onion
- ¼ cup thinly sliced fresh ginger
- 6 cloves garlic, minced
- 1 pound boneless, skinless chicken thighs, trimmed and cut into 1/2-inch pieces
- 4 cups chicken broth
- 1 ½ cups peeled and cubed green papaya or chayote
- 2 cups chopped bok choy leaves
- 1 tablespoon fish sauce
- ¼ teaspoon salt
- ¼ teaspoon ground black pepper

Heat oil in a large pot over medium heat. Add onion, ginger and garlic; cook, stirring about 3 minutes. Add chicken and broth, stirring until the chicken is just cooked through, about 5 minutes. Add papaya (or chayote),or bok choy, fish sauce, salt and pepper; continue simmering until the vegetables are cooked through - about 5 minutes.

Ladle into a bowl and enjoy!

Sharon's Versatile Soup

My friend Sharon is a wonderful cook. This soup can also be turned into a dip if you blend it.

- 1 1/2 Tlb Coconut Oil
- 1 med Onion chopped
- 1 med Jalapeno finely diced
- 3 cloves of Garlic minced
- 1 tsp Oregano
- 1 tsp Cumin
- 1 Lg Bay leaf
- 1 tsp of Sea Salt
- 1/4 tsp Pepper
- Pinch of Cayenne Pepper
- 1 lb of Red Lentils
- 32 oz of low sodium Vegetable Broth
- 1-2 cups of water (depending on how think you want the recipe to be) You can always add more water later.
- 2 Tlb of Apple Cider Vinegar
- 1 Tlb Swerve
- Juice of half a lime
- 1/4 c chopped Cilantro

In a large pot add the coconut oil and saute onion, and jalapeno for a few minutes.

Add the garlic and spices and saute for a few minutes longer. Don't burn the garlic.

Add the Vegetable broth, water, vinegar, swerve, and red lentils. Stir, bring to a boil, turn down the heat and simmer, covered for 45 min or until done.

Remove from heat and adjust seasonings.

Let it cool for about 10 min then add the lime juice and chopped cilantro. Stir.

Serve and enjoy.

Italian Spring Vegetable Soup

Another soup from Sharon Merriman

The beauty of this recipe is you don't have to use the same ingredients when it comes to the veggies.

If you don't like Kale use Spinach. It's a no go on Asparagus? Use String Beans. Don't like Shitake? Leave them out or try a different mushroom. You can even do a fridge "DUMP" with whatever veg you have hanging out as leftovers. And it comes together in about 45 min.

- 1 1/2 Tlb Olive Oil
- 1 med Onion chopped
- 2 Lg Carrots quartered and sliced
- 1 Lg stalk of Celery

- 6 cloves of Garlic minced

- 1 tsp Oregano

- 1/2 tsp Rosemary

- 1/4 tsp Thyme

- 1tsp Sea Salt

- 1/2 tsp Pepper

- 2 Bay leaves

- 4 oz Shitake mushrooms

————————————————

- 1 26oz chopped Tomatoes

- 1 c water

- 4 c Bone Broth, Vegetable Broth, or Chicken stock (unsalted or low sodium) If you use the ones with sodium leave out the salt above and adjust after to your own taste.

- 1/4 c Quinoa. I used Quinoa with Spinach by Pereg Natural Foods but you can use any Quinoa. Preferable white for aesthetics.

————————————————

- 1 med Zucchini quartered and sliced into 1/2" pieces

- 8 spears of Asparagus, cut on the diagonal into 1/2" pieces

- 1 1/2 cups of Kale, removed from the stem, chopped

- 1/2 c frozen Peas

————————————————

- 1/2 c Pecorino Romano
- 1 handful of fresh chopped Basil or Parsley.

Heat a large pot or dutch oven on med.

Add the Olive Oil, Onion, Carrots, Celery, Salt, Pepper, Oregano, Rosemary, Thyme, and Bay leaves.

Saute for 4-5 min on med low until they begin to brown. Add Garlic and mushrooms continuing to sauté for several minutes.

Add the Chopped Tomatoes, Water, Broth, and Quinoa stirring and scrubbing off the bits of brown off the bottom of the pan.

Cover and simmer on low heat for 20 min.

Uncover and add Zucchini, Asparagus, and Kale. Cover and simmer another 10 min.

Uncover and remove from heat.

Stir in the Pecorino Romano and fresh chopped herbs.

Taste for seasonings.

Serve with a sprinkle of Pecorino Romano on the top.

Enjoy.

CHAPTER SEVEN

OTHER PULSE THERAPIES

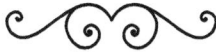

Earlier in the book we shared the research of Thomas Seyfried and his associates regarding the healing effects of the hyperbaric oxygen therapy on the mitochondria and how it is incorporated in Press-Pulse therapy. There are additional pulse methods that can be used to cleanse and replenish the body with oxygen and nutrients to alter the inner terrain in support of healing.

The Tom Tam Healing Modality

Tom Tam, a Boston-based acupuncturist combines the Warburg theory with traditional Chinese medicine for the foundation of his healing system. After arriving in the United States in 1975 as a political refugee from China, Tam established himself as a prominent acupuncturist and a practitioner in the art of traditional Chinese Medicine. At his studio in Haverhill, Massachusetts he has worked with hundreds of patients including referrals from the world-renowned hospitals in Boston. His approach has stretched across the world with doctors in Florence, Italy incorporating his methods into their cancer protocols.[41]

Among the many success stories, one involves a man diagnosed with stage four pancreatic cancer, with only a five percent chance of survival. On July 3, 2008, 11 days before his first wedding anniversary, Frank Guidara was diagnosed with pancreatic cancer. In Western medicine, pancreatic cancer is generally viewed as "not survivable".[42]

Frank underwent two weeks of chemotherapy in pill form, five days of radiation therapy, and six rounds of intravenous chemotherapy. In addition to this, he and his wife, Juliette began eating a raw food diet, and researched other therapies that supported his immune system. This led to Tam's office in Boston and a regimen of Tui Na massage. Frank is currently thriving and shows no signs of malignancy. In fact, Juliette is now a practitioner of Tam's approach.

What is Tam doing to get these kinds of results? Combining his foundational knowledge of traditional Chinese Medicine with what he has learned through treating patients, Tam has separated the body into two biological systems. He refers to these systems as the Biochemical and Bioelectrical and he believes they are the main pathways by which all cells, organs, and nerves communicate with each other. If there is a break in communication, the body cannot repair itself.[43]

The Biochemical System is the focus of Western medicine. Driven by the pharmaceutical industry, this looks at the connection between hormones and chemical reactions within the body. Tom Tam believes that doctors have overlooked the most important piece of the puzzle - the Bioelectrical System, better known as the nervous system.

The cornerstone of human physiological function is the ability to generate signals from cell to cell via the nervous system. If there is a broken or blocked circuit in the nervous system, the body cannot function normally. Tam theorizes that the dysfunction of the nervous system is mainly to blame for the development of cancer cells and the spread of disease. In fact, his research shows that just about every cancer patient has a blockage in the phrenic nerve area. Repair the damage, and function of the nerve will be restored.

The phrenic nerve is what controls the diaphragm and the diaphragm controls oxygen intake. An energy flow breakdown in the phrenic nerve means there is a reduction in the amount of oxygen uptake in the blood. Low oxygen means more potential for cancer to thrive. If a problem with the phrenic nerve is a leading contributor to cancer, how does Tam's method fix this problem?

The Importance of Healthy Nervous System Function

The nervous system is divided into two parts – central and peripheral. The central nervous system consists of the brain and the spinal cord. The peripheral nervous system carries signals throughout the entire body, including all internal organs.

From there, the peripheral system is divided further into two more groups the somatic nervous system and the autonomic nervous system. The somatic nervous system is considered to be voluntary, meaning that it can be controlled by the conscious mind, such as blinking your eye, or waving your hand.

The autonomic system governs all organ functions and controls involuntary muscle response such as the beating of the heart and breathing. It is divided even further into two more parts - the sympathetic and the parasympathetic nervous systems. The sympathetic nervous system controls the fight or flight responses, and the parasympathetic system is responsible for rest and digest.[44]

A blockage, or a high resistance of energy flow, in the autonomic system can cause a problem with the signals passing through it from the brain. When an organ has an energy blockage coming from its autonomic nerve, it results in a lack of oxygen uptake in that particular organ. Anything from breathing, heart rate, digestion, urination, perspiration, and hormone production can be affected by a malfunction in this system.

Western medicine has proven that bioelectrical waves flow freely throughout the body. Brain waves are measured through EEG (electroencephalogram), and the strength of the heart is measured through EKG (electrocardiogram) waves, so we know the bioelectrical energy flow is real and true. In cancer patients the phrenic nerve, which runs down either side of the neck and down through the torso, ending at the diaphragm, will always have an energy blockage.

Fixing The Phrenic Nerve With Tui Na

For centuries, the people of China have used the energy of therapeutic touch to facilitate healing of specific parts of the body. Tui Na is a type of acupressure massage designed to stimulate certain energy pathways called meridians. These meridians are made up of a series of key points which create a circuit board controlling the ebb and flow of life force called Qi, or Chi. Each meridian has its own grouping of energy points which connect to each other in a circuit.[45]

In Traditional Chinese Medicine (TCM), chi is the electromagnetic energy which flows through all living things, and it is used as a measurement of vitality. In TCM theory there are fourteen different meridians which are named after specific organs. It is important to maintain the flow of energy if you want a healthy body. A dysfunctional phrenic nerve means an interruption in energy flow.

The phrenic nerve radiates from cervical spinal nerve points C3, C4, and C5 - located in the neck. The reflex point is in the LI-17 (large intestine meridian) vicinity, located near both collar bones. When a blockage is detected in those areas the cancer patient will feel acute pain.

To fix this blockage, Tam stimulates the specific correlating areas along the spine to reconnect lost energy pathways by using the Tui Na massage. If there is no Tui Na practitioner in your area, any massage therapist trained in acupressure point massage will know how to stimulate the LI-17 pressure point.[46]

The Spinal Column and Raindrop Therapy

In my first book about cancer, *"Essential Oils And Cancer: How To Effectively Use The Right Essential Oils To Confuse And Kill Cancer Cells"*, I share the daily ritual I performed on my brother's spine during his bout with prostate cancer. This technique is loosely based on a healing ritual called Raindrop Therapy. I discovered this approach from reading about Gary Young's (Young Living Essential Oils founder) experience learning healing methods from a Native American medicine man of the Lakota Tribe.

Raindrop Therapy involves dropping small amounts of specific essential oils, one-by-one, onto the spinal column and massaging them into the sides of the spine. I often wondered, why the spine? Now I know.

Each section of the spinal cord correlates with specific areas of the body. When the entire spinal column is stimulated, the whole sympathetic nervous system also becomes stimulated. This allows bioelectricity to flow once again to areas that were blocked.

In addition to restoring bioelectrical flow to the spine, the combination of essential oils and massage help to relieve the spinal area of inflammation, viral and bacterial remnants, and infections. By reducing any swelling that may be happening along the spinal column, blood flow and energy flow are improved throughout the nervous system. The massage also helps to minimize spinal misalignments, leading to a positive effect on the damaged phrenic nerve area.

What Are Essential Oils?

Essential oils are the concentrated volatile oils distilled from various parts of a plant and can come from the seed, root, stem, leaf, bark, sap, or flower. The oils contain specific chemical constituents which have a beneficial effect on the immune system. Different plant species contain different levels of different constituents.

For instance, Frankincense essential oil is distilled from the hardened sap (resin) of the olibanum tree which grows mainly in the Middle East. The oil is best known as one of the three gifts given to Jesus Christ at the time of his birth by three wise men, but recently the oil has been used by cancer patients for its medicinal purposes. Frankincense has certain cancer-fighting organic compounds called, terpenes. Among them are alpha-pinene, alpha-amyrin, beta-amyrin, beta-phellandrene, and camphene. This terpene cocktail has proven effective in killing cancer cells in recent studies[47].

These compounds can be introduced into the bloodstream by way of spinal massage. There is also the added benefit of aromatherapy, which naturally causes a reduction in stress hormones such as cortisol. Doing this ritual on a daily basis is ideal. Here's how you can do it.

How To Conduct A Spinal Massage

My book, *"Essential Oils and Cancer: How to Effectively Use the Right Essential Oils to Confuse and Kill Cancer Cells"* has a list of essential oils that are proven to be effective for each specific type of cancer ranging from breast cancer to prostate cancer. All the lists contain Frankincense. Please make sure to use oils of higher quality. The label will often say "therapeutic grade".

If you are fortunate enough to have a licensed practitioner trained to give Raindrop Therapy you can schedule a weekly appointment. Please make sure the therapist uses the correct essential oils that are designated for the cancer you have. If you cannot find a practitioner, or you cannot afford one, you can do your own spinal massage similar to Raindrop with the help of a friend.

After gathering your essential oils, find a comfortable place to lie face down. Lying down is much better than standing up. If you're new to using essential oils you should use them diluted in a carrier oil. A carrier oil is any kind of oil used to dilute essential oils and "carry" it to the skin. Fractionated coconut oil, grapeseed oil, and jojoba oil are all wonderful choices for carrier oils. Dilute the oil at least 5:1. For the more intense oils like clove and oregano, please use a diffuser to breathe in the essential oil particles instead of applying them directly onto the skin. Clove and oregano may burn the skin.

Begin by dropping each oil individually, one by one, along either side of the spine starting from the base of the neck all the way down to the small of the back. Hold the bottle at least one foot above the spine and let one drop fall an inch to the right of the cervical spine (neck area), then slowly move down and let another drop fall an inch to the left. Continue to move all the way down the spine in a zig-zag motion. Next, in a clockwise motion, massage the oil into the areas where you dropped them. There should be 8-10 drops total. Repeat this with the next oil on the list until complete.

After you are done you can have your helper cover the area with a warm moist towel to open the pores and help push the essential oils further into the spinal area. For further instructions you can refer to my book "Essential Oils and Cancer".

Ozone Therapy

Ozone is both a natural and man-made gas composed of three oxygen atoms with the chemical name O3. It is a highly reactive gas that occurs naturally in the Earth's upper atmosphere and in 1896 Nikola Tesla patented the first ozone generator. Since then, ozone has been used medically for over 100 years.

During the First World War, German doctors discovered that O3 possessed antibacterial properties and used it to aid wound recovery. They found that it not only remedied infections, but it also had anti-inflammatory qualities. Over sixty years later, in the late 1980's, German physicians used ozone intravenously on HIV patients. This treatment, known as major auto-hemotransfusion, involves extracting blood from an IV inserted in the patient's arm and then running it through an ozone gas generator. The blood is disinfected and becomes saturated with oxygen before it is re-injected back into the bloodstream. The team found that the gas was very effective in disinfecting and oxygenating the blood to the point where viruses could not survive.

Major autohemotranfusion was subsequently used in a 2004 pilot study in Hamburg, Germany to determine the impact on cancer patients and the potential to reverse hypoxia in cancer tumors. This study was built on the idea that chemotherapy and radiation treatment depend on the presence of oxygen in the blood and within the tumor. Over the course of one week, 18 patients were given ozone treatment every other day. At the conclusion of the study, the team found a significant decrease in hypoxic areas overall. When the patients were individually assessed, the findings showed the highest positive impact on tumors most deprived of oxygen.[48]

Key Takeaways and Action Steps

- Using his knowledge of Traditional Chinese Medicine, acupuncturist Tom Tam found that cancer patients have pain and bioelectrical energy blockages along the phrenic nerve.

- The phrenic nerve is responsible for the movement of the diaphragm which controls oxygen intake.

- The phrenic nerve can be manipulated by using TuiNa medical massage.

CHAPTER EIGHT

PRESS PULSE PRACTITIONERS & PATIENT STORIES

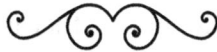

The press-pulse therapeutic strategy for cancer management is far more than just a theory, scientific methodology, or a series of clinical tests. It is also being used by people right now in their battle against cancer. In this chapter, I'll share the real-world stories of three people who used the press-pulse approach to fight back and the practitioners who helped them.

Dr. Colin E. Champ[49]

Dr. Colin E. Champ is a board certified (American Board of Radiology) Radiation Oncologist and practices at the Duke Cancer Center in Durham, North Carolina. A native of Pittsburgh, PA, he grew up in a tight-knit Southern Italian family with a grandfather who served as the inspiration and motivation for his career choice. His grandfather had his own organic vegetable garden with organic fertilizer well before either of those things became a health craze. Dr. Champ studied chemical engineering at the Massachusetts Institute of Technology (MIT) and has been a dedicated proponent of fitness since his youth.

After trying his hand at financial consulting, his passion for health and exercise led him to Jefferson Medical College in Philadelphia, receiving his degree there and getting accepted into their competitive residency training program. In the years since, he has co-hosted a podcast that is top-ranked in the US, England, and Australia; been featured in the Boston Globe; Sanjay Gupta's *The Gupta Guide*, the National Cancer Institute at the National Institute of Health, and the American Society of Clinical Oncology. In 2014, he released his first book, "*Misguided Medicine: The truth behind ill-advised medical recommendations and how to take health back into your hands.*"

On his website, Dr. Champ states that "...while curing people of cancer is the #1 part of his job, the ability to show people how healthier choices can help keep the cancer away as well as get them feeling better for decades down the road is a strong second." With strong indicators about the effects of the ketogenic diet on "starving" existing cancer cells of the glucose they crave so heavily, Dr. Champ began to investigate whether a combination of diet and fasting could also play a role in preventing cancer from occurring in the first place. Going through nearly a century of data and looking at a number of diets, Dr. Champ has shown that not only is a low-carb diet one of the best cancer prevention strategies, it enhances the effectiveness of radiation therapy during cancer treatment while protecting healthy cells.

Miriam Kalamian[50]

Miriam Kalamian is board certified in nutrition (CNS) by the Board for Certification of Nutrition Specialists and has a Master of Education (EdM) from Smith College and a Master of Human Nutrition (MS) from Eastern Michigan University. Her story is not of her professional accomplishments, but of a personal challenge and a mother's unwavering devotion. This is the story of Miriam's 4-year-old son Raffi.

The Kalamians adopted Raffi as a toddler. Both parents and a child psychologist thought he suffered from attachment disorder. He was malnourished prior to his adoption and an eye exam revealed he had rickets and a condition called optic nerve pallor. Raffi struggled with focus and was unable to be away from his mother for even a few minutes. Erring on the side of caution, the doctor decided to have an MRI done on his brain to rule out abnormalities. When the Kalamians got the call, the pediatrician told her that there was a large tumor in his brain and Raffi needed to get to a children's hospital right away. This meant a 16-hour drive through a blizzard and surgery the next day for a biopsy. It was Christmas Eve 2004.

Raffi's mother and father went "all-in" on the treatments and procedures to try to help their son fight off the monster growing inside of him. Raffi underwent three surgeries and multiple rounds of chemotherapy and various medications. None of those worked and within two years, their son was steadily losing the battle to his tumor. His vision was suffering. His language skills deteriorated at an age where those of his peers were rapidly advancing. His motor skills were downgrading as well, and he was suffering endocrine problems that were significantly affecting his vital functions.

In March 2007, the Kalamians learned about Dr. Thomas Seyfried and the press-pulse therapy method. Miriam discovered Dr. Seyfried's work soon after his findings about the impact of the ketogenic diet on cancer were published.

Raffi's parents were dedicated to making the treatment possible for their son, so they started looking for safe environments. Johns Hopkins Hospital, which had a history of safely implementing the same type of diet for children with serious epilepsy, became the answer. The team at Johns Hopkins had written a book about the topic of ketogenic diets making it a perfect environment. Miriam didn't stop with the book, she wanted to know the science supporting it from top to bottom. That same year she applied to, and was accepted into, Eastern Michigan University's Master of Science program for Human Nutrition.

The Kalamians met with Raffi's pediatrician and oncologist to discuss giving the press-pulse method a chance. The doctors got on board, but didn't want to only follow the diet, so they agreed to a low-dose chemotherapy drug coupled with the new nutritional plan. Raffi had taken the same drug at higher doses the previous year with no results.

Three months after the beginning the combined protocol, an MRI showed results that no one on the team could have dreamed of - Raffi's tumor shrunk by 15%. The ketogenic method was succeeding where every conventional therapy had failed. Over the next three years, Raffi continued the ketogenic diet and eventually the pediatrician and oncologist agreed that chemotherapy was not required. Raffi continued to get regular MRIs and clinical visits. The tumor did not disappear altogether, but it reduced in size enough for doctors to term it "essentially stable". Little by little, Raffi began to reverse some of the devastating effects that the tumor had stripped away from the normal life of an active little boy. He was not in full remission and there were still problems inside of his body, but he moved well past the initial 5-year life expectancy.

In 2010, Raffi got to celebrate with his mother when she earned her Master's in Human Nutrition. The family got more time with each other than anyone could have dreamed of back in December 2004 when doctors first delivered the devastating news. Ultimately, Raffi lost his fight on April 17, 2013. A large inoperable cyst had appeared on his brainstem, and complications from it took his life at age 13. In large part to the ketogenic diet and the press-pulse therapy plan, he exceeded the best life expectancy predictions by more than five years.

Invested in her son's battle and so moved by an alternative approach, Miriam joined Dietary Therapies LLC as a nutrition educator, consultant, and author. Tailoring the ketogenic diet to meet the needs cancer patients has become her focus and passion. In 2017, she wrote "*Keto for Cancer: Ketogenic Metabolic Therapy as a Targeted Nutritional Strategy*". The foreword for her book was written by Dr. Thomas Seyfried.

Four years after Raffi passed, Miriam did a TedX talk advocating for a therapeutic ketogenic diet. She spoke of Raffi undergoing 14 straight months of aggressive chemotherapy, none of which worked to slow the tumor at all. She talked about the six different opinions from six different oncology centers on what to do next; including one who suggested stopping all treatment attempts and just "letting him go". Another wanted to conduct multiple invasive surgeries to try and take the tumor out entirely.

She tells of how she was terrified to try the diet with the pediatrician and the oncologist monitoring him throughout. Raffi loved pasta, but that is one of the highest carb-count foods, so they replaced it with spaghetti squash and zucchini strips - the same texture and look as pasta for a young boy. The bread of sandwiches was transitioned out and sliced meat roll ups became the new craze. Quiches and keto muffins were the new baked goods in the household. Healthy fats made their way into almost anything he ate in the form of butter and cream and coconut oil. When he wanted something crunchy, macadamia nuts were the snack of choice. When he wanted something creamy, it was time to open an avocado.

As a proponent of the ketogenic diet, Miriam Kalamian is still meeting resistance as she writes her books, gives interviews, and meets with parents and physicians who are curious enough to ask aboutit as an alternative or a supplement to their current therapies. When these people ask for proof, she has the ultimate ace in the hole, she lived the proof. She can show them a gorgeous photo of Raffi smiling ear to ear, bundled up and riding his bicycle in the snow at an age when most kids with brain tumors can't do much better than seeing snow out the window of the hospital room. She advocates that it's not necessary to wait for clinical trials to try the ketogenic diet for yourself if you have cancer, and traditional methods are not helping you. She jokes that if your doctor says that your diet is not important, he's just given you the go-ahead to try ketogenic.

Miriam Kalamian is a realist. She tells the people she interacts with that you can't hide from cancer. If it's not coming for you, it's going to come for someone you love. What you can do is get ready to fight it when it arrives with the best possible combination of weapons and strategies. Like Dr. Champ, Miriam is a strong proponent for starting the ketogenic diet well before you get a diagnosis. The fewer carbs, the fewer potential free radicals that could turn into tumors. The sooner you start, the more likely you are to beat cancer to the punch and keep it out of your system altogether.

Maggie Jones[51]

You might question Maggie Jones' sanity when you read her opening statement: *"Terminal cancer is the best thing that ever happened to me"*. Not many people are capable of saying that, because let's be honest, if you get terminal cancer it means the end of the road is coming much sooner than you would probably like. However, Jones is one of those unique people that not only make this book special, but also make the press-pulse therapy plan such an amazing thing to learn about.

When Jones turned 40, she and her husband decided to go all-out with the adventure of a lifetime, a trip to Hong Kong from their home in Los Angeles. A month later Jones was undergoing a very different sort of adventure, also something she had never encountered, but an adventure she would not have wished on her worst enemy. After the trip she started having terrible pain and symptoms that made no sense for someone with her fairly spotless family medical history. Nobody closely related had ever suffered from cancer and she didn't smoke. And yet she was struggling to breathe and getting pain all over her body.

Clearly something was wrong with her, but when the diagnosis came back it caused total disbelief for Jones and her husband. She had terminal lung cancer that had rapidly spread to her eye, her brain, and more than a dozen of her lymph nodes, followed shortly thereafter by her liver and abdomen. It was like cancer had been injected into her body and spread like fire through a paper factory. As if the 'C' word wasn't bad enough, her doctor followed up with a devastating 1-2 combination punch. The median survival time with conventional treatment was six-to-eight months, meaning they were not expecting her to see her 41st birthday. The five-year survival rate for the combination of cancers and the severity of it all was 0%.

While she didn't appear unhealthy, Jones would soon learn that she had been setting herself up for a visit from the 'C' word for years. It started with the huge helpings of stress she was serving up day after day in her job as a corporate executive providing the only source of income for her family. She ate what she calls the standard American diet, but almost never exercised, other than raising a wine glass to her lips. Her body was full of inflammation from the stress and the lack of exercise, and she didn't even know it. No one who knew her would call her anywhere close to overweight, but she was closer to the clinical definition of it than she felt comfortable with. She looked like the typical American 9-to-5er.

With quite literally nothing to lose, she decided that if medicine couldn't fight the cancerous forces ravaging her body from the inside out, she would have to take control of the battlefield herself. She didn't waste precious time feeling sorry for herself, instead she got to work doing research on what she could do to give herself a chance at fighting back.

It started with a therapeutic water fast to shock the body into using its fat stores to power its mechanics. When the fast was over, she made a promise to herself that when she started eating again, the only food that would go into her body would be something that could heal her body, along with the medicine the doctors had prescribed. Over the next six months, she ate strictly from an approved whole food, plant-based ketogenic diet. Six months was the minimum amount of time she had left to live according to the diagnosis. In those six months, she lost more than 50 pounds of fat and found herself back to a true healthy weight for the first time since her childhood.

As she was fighting off hunger pangs and letting the world know that she was not quite dead yet, she started learning more and more about the intimate, connected relationship between stress, cancer, and inflammation. She realized her constant states of stress and inflammation had directly contributed to how quickly the cancer had spread and how thoroughly it had taken over her body. She countered these effects with an eight-week course in stress reduction that was based on being mindful of your surroundings, how you're feeling, what things you're letting control your emotions, etc. She had never attempted yoga or meditation in her entire life, but now took to them like a fish to water, finding them the perfect release for all of her worries and doubts about what the future had in store for her. She was able to view her body beyond the physical and recognize it as a culmination of the physical, mental, emotional, and spiritual parts of her life.

At the time of her diagnosis, Jones could not sleep lying down because her lungs were constantly filling with cancerous fluid. She was mostly blind in her right eye. She had confusing episodes brought on by a vicious combination of brain radiation, chemotherapy and the presence of multiple brain tumors.

A year passed - the year that she was supposed to have died in. However, Jones found herself in the best physical condition of her life. She went back to work. Slowly at first, and then full time. She filled her weekends with long hikes instead of cocktails. At night she took yoga classes instead of picking up that wine glass. Her relationship with her husband evolved and strengthened. She connected with her family in ways she never had before. Food and alcohol were no longer viewed as rewards. Her whole lifestyle changed and she was infinitely happier as a result. A year after her terminal diagnosis, Jones had no evidence of active cancer in her body. The tumors remain, but they are remarkably smaller.

Jones now runs her own blog on CancerV.me in which she gives frequent updates as well as informing others on the power of the ketogenic diet, getting the right amount of exercise, and what various research and advancements are being made in the ketogenic field. In her June 2020 medical update, she reported that her blood markers remain in the normal range, meaning the cancer has not reactivated despite the continued presence of the tumors in her body. She continues to take the cancer drug TKI and has developed overt hypothyroidism as a result, but it corresponds with improved outcomes in cancer treatment, which means that things are going well on the inside.

One of the most appreciated things she does on her blog is provide ketogenic-friendly recipes to other cancer sufferers. One of the biggest burdens for people suffering cancer badly enough to where ketogenic diets become an approved technique is figuring out what to eat, how much to eat, and when to eat. When you've been overweight or obese your whole life and you're suddenly told to eat a completely different diet, and oh by the way you also have cancer, people tend to try to change their tune but end up going back to their old ways as frustration mounts on what they can eat and what recipes make sense for their new lifestyle.

Jones does not think that the cancer will not return. She suspects it will still defeat her at some point, probably younger than a normal person would like. It does not bother her, however, as she believes that in the time since her diagnosis, she has lived more richly and deeply than in most of the years before she was diagnosed.

She calls cancer the messenger that woke her up to the terrible way she was living and got her back on the right path, not just in terms of health and nutrition, but in terms of her lifestyle, her relationships ,and her spirituality. She does not refer to herself as a cancer survivor, but rather as a cancer thriver.

Judy Seeger, ND[52]

By the time she was 18 years old, Judy Seeger was in the worst shape of her life. Poor dietary choices left her suffering from chronic fatigue, migraine headaches, constant sinus infections, dizzy spells and constipation. Growing up in New York City with European parents, Judy admits she had a sweet tooth. Fresh fruits and vegetables were hard to come by, so instead she opted for white bread and peanut butter and jelly sandwiches. She shudders to think of what might have happened to her health had she continued down that path.

Thankfully, in 1978 Judy was introduced to the power of cleansing and natural detoxification, a path that would ultimately lead to healing and self-discovery. She was fortunate enough to be trained by world-renowned healers like master herbalist, Dr. John Christopher, and nutritionist, Dr. Bernard Jensen.

But it was her mentor, Dr. Joel Robbins, MD, DC, ND who really influenced her eating and thinking habits. She began to live a life of peace, let go of anger, and embraced the mentality of healing the whole body, mind and spirit. Judy became a naturopathic physician, and after over 35 years of experience she has become one of the leading experts on cancer detoxification using ozone therapy in the United States. At her practice based out of the West Palm Beach area in Florida, she has educated hundreds of other practitioners and patients on the benefits of using ozone therapy as part of the cancer-fighting toolbox. Judy not only applied ozone therapy to target her fight against Lyme disease, but has applied it to hundreds of her patients.

As previously mentioned in the last chapter, ozone therapy has been used for decades, beginning in Europe, to correct many health issues. Problems such as bacterial overgrowth, viruses, fungal infections, yeast and mold can be addressed through ozone exposure. Simultaneously, it strengthens cell walls and helps reactivate the immune system by stimulating white blood cell production. By increasing the amount of oxygen in the blood, cell respiration is normalized, and lactic acid build up is reduced which are both beneficial to fighting cancer.

On Judy's website (judyseegerdetox.com) she explains how to realize the benefits of using ozone safely from your home. You can download a free guide on five ways ozone can be used at home to kill pathogens. Like Dr Seyfried and Dr. Champ, Dr. Seeger believes that the key to complete recovery from cancer is not dependent upon one therapy only, but by using an array of many treatments simultaneously to kill the disease.

BEAUTY COUNTER INFO

Finally, before we end the book, lets talk about the importance of "clean" products on your face and body.....

There are so many reasons to switch to cleaner products. Maybe you have concerns about how your personal-care products might be negatively impacting your health. Or your children's health. Or the environment. Perhaps you're just tired of buying skin care products that don't do what they claim. Whatever your reasons let me introduce you to Beautycounter.

Beautycounter develops and distributes its own high-performing products made with ingredients significantly safer for health — including skin-care, color cosmetics, advanced anti-aging, kids, baby, men's and personal-care collections — all while driving a growing national movement to demand better regulations for the beauty industry.

Since its launch in 2013, Beautycounter has attracted national attention as the first brand to take a meaningful position on cosmetic reform. Through its trademarked The Never List™, Beautycounter has prohibited the use of more than 1,800 questionable or harmful ingredients in their product formulations, well beyond the 30 banned by U.S. law. Beautycounter also works extensively at the federal level to improve transparency and accountability of the beauty industry, and advocates for stronger cosmetic safety laws which have stood largely unchanged since 1938. In December 2019, Gregg Renfrew was invited to testify as an expert witness before Congress in only the second hearing on cosmetic reform held in the House in the past 40 years. Speaking for millions of Americans, Renfrew delivered a powerful message: the FDA must better protect consumers, and the time to act is now.

Did you know?

The average man uses around six skincare products per day, the average female uses around twelve.

Conventical skincare and especially makeup is often high in heavy metals! This is particularly a problem with many "natural" makeups. Most conventional lipstick is also high in lead, and the half-life of lead in the body can be up to 30 years. That means every time you put on some lipstick, you might be putting some lead into your bones, which might not leave for three decades.

For more information on how you can clean up your and your family's daily skin care routines visit:

beautycounter.com/SharonMerriman

SOURCES

- https://www.amazon.com/Keto-Cancer-Ketogenic-Metabolic-Nutritional/dp/1603587012?SubscriptionId=AKIAIOCEBIGP6NUBL47A&tag=dietarytherap-20&linkCode=xm2&camp=2025&creative=165953&creativeASIN=1603587012

- https://www.dietarytherapies.com/introduction

- http://www.ketoforcancer.org/Raffi_s_Story.html

- https://www.youtube.com/watch?v=zYcjnGi5cOs

- https://thriveglobal.com/stories/why-terminal-cancer-is-the-best-thing-that-ever-happened-to-me/

- https://cancerv.me/author/magzillaj0nes/#:~:text=Maggie%20Jones-,Maggie%20Jones,every%20moment%20of%20this%20life.

ACKNOWLEDGEMENTS

A huge debt of gratitude is owed to the team who made this book possible. Thank you to my editor, Michelle Addario. There's no doubt you've made this book better with your sharp eye and your hard work behind the scenes. You've spent countless hours making sure everything was right. Steven Fraser, my junior editor, I appreciate your work as well. Your patience and your friendship means everything to me.

Thank you to Jessica Bell Design for my beautiful cover (I love it). Also a big hug of gratitude goes to Sharon Merriman who has been invaluable to me. Your recipes are fabulous and our upcoming cookbook for Lifechanger is something I look forward to.

Last but not least, I'd like to thank Mark Michaud from Blue Road Consulting in Boston. From start to finish you believed in my project and provided the encouragement that was needed to get things done. Thank you so much.

NOTES

1   Cancer Research UK, "People Fear Cancer More Than Any Other
    Disease" August 16, 2011
    Healthcare Global.com "Survey Reveals Cancer Is Most Feared Disease"
    August 15, 2020

2   E.H. Rosenbaum, MD, I. Sadora, and R. Rosenbaum, MA, Stanford
    Center for Integrative Medicine. med.stanford.edu/survivingcancer/
    cancers-existential-questions/cancer-will-to-live.html Stanford
    Medicine 2020

3   H. Elrod "What I Did To Beat Cancer" HalElrod.com

4   Dana Farber Cancer Institute Dana-Farber.org

5   "On The Antiquity Of Cancer" PLOS ONE 2014; 9(3);e90924
    Published online 2014 March 2017 doi 10.1371/journal.pone.0090924

6   T.N. Seyfried "Cancer As A Mitochondrial Metabolic Disease" Front
    Cell Dev. Biology 2015; 3:43 US National Library of Medicine

7   R.G. McKinnell "The Lucke Frog Kidney Tumor And Its Herpes Virus"
    Dept. of Zoology, University of Minnesota, Minneapolis
    American Zoology, 13:97-114 (1973)

8   Beatrice Mintz "Simian Virus 40 DNA Sequences In DNA of Healthy
    Adult Mice Derived From Preimplantation Blastocysts Injected With
    Viral DNA" Proc. Natl. Acad. Sci. USA 71(4): 1250-4
    Adam R. Navis "The Embryo Project Encyclopedia" pub: 2009-01-21

9   Somatic Mutation - NIH: National Cancer Institute cancer.gov/
    publications/dictionaries/cancer-terms/def/somatic-mutation
    Adam R. Navis "The Embryo Project Encyclopedia" pub: 2009-01-21

10 L. Li, M.C. Connelly, C. Wetmore, T. Curran, J.I. Morgan "Mouse Embryos Cloned for Brain Tumors" AACR Publications June 2003 Dept. of Developmental Neurobiology, St. Jude's Children's Research Hospital, Memphis, Tenn.

11 NIH: National Human Genome Research Institute www.genome.gov/ human-genome-project
The Cancer Genome Atlas www.cancerresearchfdn.org/young-investigator-george-souroullas 02-25-2019

12 Y. Zhang, J. Park, T. Lee, P. Yotnda, W. Chan, C. Creighton, B.A. Kaipparettu, L. Wong "Crosstalk from Non-Cancerous Mitochondria Can Inhibit Tumor Properties of Metastatic Cells by Suppressing Oncogenic Pathways"
Medicine, Biology PLOS ONE Journal. pone. 0061747 Corpus ID: 14204144 published 2013

13 M. V. Liberti, J.W. Locasale "The Warburg Effect: How Does It Benefit Cancer Cells" Trends Biochem Sci PMC 2017 March 1
Published online: 2016 Jan 5 doi 10 1016/j.tibs.2015.12.001

14 G. Zuccoli, N. Marcello, A Pisanello, F. Servadei, S. Vaccaro, P. Mukherjee, T. N. Seyfried Human Trial "Metabolic Management of Glioblastoma Multiforme Using Standard Therapy Together With a Restricted Ketogenic Diet" Nutrition & Metabolism (Lond) 2010; 7:33 PMCID: PMC2874558

15 Journal: Current Oncology, 2015 Aug. 22

16 NDSS: "Steroid Medications and Diabetes Facts" ndss.com.au/about-diabetes/resources/find-a-resource
"Steroids May Affect Your Blood Sugar Level" 2018 March www.abta.org

17 Hindawi "Ketogenic Diet in Neuromuscular and Neurodegenerative Diseases"
Biomed Research International 2014 Article ID 474296

18 Human Trial "Efficacy of Metabolically Supported Chemotherapy Combined with Ketogenic Diet, Hyperthermia, and Hyperbaric Oxygen Therapy for Stage IV Triple-Negative Breast Cancer" World Cancer Research Fund American Institute for Cancer Research

19   Human Trial "Feasibility, Safety, and Beneficial Effects of MCT Oil-
     Based Ketogenic Diet for Breast Cancer Treatment: A Randomized
     Controlled Trial Study" NIH National Library of Medicine National
     Center for Biotechnology Info PubMed.gov Nutr. Cancer, 2020; 72 (4):
     627-634, doi: 10.1080/01635581.2019 Epub 2019 Sept. 9

20   Jocelyn Tan-Shalaby, MD "Ketogenic Diets and Emerging Evidence"
     NCBI US Natl. Library of Medicine Natl. Institute of Health
     Federal Practitioner 2017 February; 34 (Suppl 1) : 37S-42S

21   C. Hicks "Short History of Fasting" Target Health, LLC Clinical
     Research June 5, 2017

22   A.M. Poff, C. Ari, P. Arnold, T.N. Seyfried, D.P. D'Agostino "Ketone
     Supplementation Decreases Tumor Cell Viability and Prolongs Survival
     of Mice With Metastatic Cancer" Wiley Intl. Journal of Cancer 2014
     Oct. 1; 135(7): 1711-1720 Published online: 2014 doi: 10.1002/ijc.28809

23   "MCT Oil 101: A Review of Medium Chain Triglycerides" Healthline.
     com/nutrition/mct-oil-101#what-it-is

24   https://highintensityhealth.com/174-angela-poff-phd-cancer-a-
     metabolic-disease-the-ketogenic-diet-warburg-effect/

25   Etan Orgel, MD, MS and Steven D. Mittelman, MD, PhD. "The Links
     Between Insulin Resistance, Diabetes, and Cancer" HHS Public Access
     Curr. Diab Rep. 2013 April 13 (2) : 213-222 doi: 10.1007/s11892-012-
     0356-6

26   The Women's Health Initiative https://www.whi.org

27   Eric C. Woolf, Nelofer Syed, and Adrienn C. Scheck "Tumor
     Metabolism, the Ketogenic Diet, and Beta-Hydroxybutyrate: Novel
     Approaches to Adjuvant Brain Tumor Therapy" Frontiers in Molecular
     Neuroscience 2016; 9: 122
     Published online: 2016 Nov 16. doi: 10.3389/fnmol.2016.00122

28   C.E Champ, J.D. Palmer, J.S. Volek, J. Glass, L. Kim, W. Shi, M. Werner-
     Wasik, D.W. Andrews, J.J. Evans "Targeting Metabolism With a
     Ketogenic Diet During Treatment of Glioblastoma Multiforme"
     Neuro-Oncology 2014 March 117(1): 125-31 doi: 10.1007/s11060-014-
     13620 Epub: 2014 Jan 19

29   J.C. Newman & E. Verdin "Ketone Bodies as Signaling Metabolites"
     Journal List HS Author Manuscript PMC 4176946   Trends
     Endocrinology Metabolism 2014 Jan: 25(1) 42-52

30   PLoS One. 2013; 8(6): e65522.
     Published online 2013 Jun 5. doi: 10.1371/journal.pone.0065522
     PMCID: PMC3673985
     PMID: 23755243
     "The Ketogenic Diet and Hyperbaric Oxygen Therapy Prolong Survival
     in Mice with Systemic Metastatic Cancer"
     Angela M. Poff, 1 , * Csilla Ari, 1 Thomas N. Seyfried, 2 and Dominic P.
     D'Agostino

31   Yun-Hee Youm 1, Kim Y Nguyen 1, Ryan W Grant 2, Emily L Goldberg
     1, Monica Bodogai 3, Dongin Kim 4, Dominic D'Agostino 5, Noah
     Planavsky 6, Christopher Lupfer 7, Thirumala D Kanneganti 7, Seokwon
     Kang 8, Tamas L Horvath 1, Tarek M Fahmy 4, Peter A Crawford 9,
     Arya Biragyn 3, Emad Alnemri 8, Vishwa Deep Dixit 10
     "The Ketone Metabolite β-hydroxybutyrate Blocks NLRP3
     Inflammatory Disease"
     Nat Med. 2015 Mar;21(3):263-9. doi: 10.1038/nm.3804. Epub 2015
     Feb.16

32   Targeting Cancer Metabolism with Ketosis and Hyperbaric Oxygen By
     Angela Marie Poff

33   Molecular Metabolism Vol. 33 March 2020 pages 102-121

34   Studies and Citations On HBOT
     Combination ketogenic diet, ketone supplementation, and hyperbaric
     oxygen therapy inhibits metastatic spread, slows tumor growth, and
     increases survival time in mice with metastatic cancer (123.7)
     Angela Poff, Nathan Ward, Thomas Seyfried, and Dominic D'Agostino
     Published Online:1 Apr 2014Abstract Number:123.7
     Scholar Commons Citation
     Poff, Angela M., "Targeting Cancer Metabolism with Ketosis and
     Hyperbaric Oxygen" (2014). Graduate Theses and Dissertations. https://
     scholarcommons.usf.edu/etd/5294

35   Tan-Shalaby, Jocelyn MD "Ketogenic Diets and Cancer: Emerging
     Evidence"
     Fed Pract. 2017 Feb; 34(Suppl 1): 37S–42S. PMCID: PMC6375425
     PMID: 30766299

36   Calorie Consumption Data - Food and Agriculture Organization of the
     United Nations 2017
     Tech 05/10/2017 "Six Charts That Show How Much More Americans
     Eat Than They Used To"

37   Biomol Ther (Seoul). 2018 Jan; 26(1): 19–28.
     Published online 2017 Dec 7. doi: 10.4062/biomolther.2017.178
     PMCID: PMC5746034
     PMID: 29212303
     Targeting Glutamine Metabolism for Cancer Treatment
     Yeon-Kyung Choi and Keun-Gyu Park*
     Molecular Metabolism
     Volume 33, March 2020, Pages 102-121
     Review
     Ketogenic diet in the treatment of cancer – Where do we stand?
     Author links open overlay panel
     Daniela D.WeberSepidehAminzadeh-GohariJuliaTulipanLucaCatalano
     René G.FeichtingerBarbaraKofler

38   Siyuan Xia,1 Ruiting Lin,1 Lingtao Jin,1 Liang Zhao,1 Hee-Bum
     Kang,1 Yaozhu Pan,1 Shuangping Liu,1 Guoqing Qian,1 Zhiyu Qian,1
     Evmorfia Konstantakou,1 Baotong Zhang,1 Jin-Tang Dong,1 Young
     Rock Chung,3 Omar Abdel-Wahab,3 Taha Merghoub,3 Lu Zhou,4
     Ragini R. Kudchadkar,1 David H. Lawson,1 Hanna J. Khoury,1 Fadlo
     R. Khuri,1 Lawrence H. Boise,1 Sagar Lonial,1 Benjamin H. Lee,5 Brian
     P. Pollack,6,7 Jack L. Arbiser,6,7 Jun Fan,2,8 Qun-Ying Lei,4,8 and Jing
     Chen1,8,9
     "Prevention of dietary fat-fueled ketogenesis attenuates BRAF V600E
     tumor growth" Cell Metab. Author manuscript; available in PMC 2018
     Feb 7.
     Published in final edited form as:
     Cell Metab. 2017 Feb 7; 25(2): 358–373.
     Published online 2017 Jan 12. doi: 10.1016/j.cmet.2016.12.010
     PMCID: PMC5299059
     NIHMSID: NIHMS838795
     PMID: 28089569

39   Francesca Consoli,1 Gianluca Barbieri,2 Matteo Picciolini,2 Daniela
     Medicina,3 Mattia Bugatti,3 Valeria Tovazzi,1 Barbara Liserre,4 Claudia
     Zambelli,3 Fausto Zorzi,4 Alfredo Berruti,1,5 Emanuele Giurisato,6,7
     and William Vermi1,8,9,*
     "A Rare Complex BRAF Mutation Involving Codon V600 and K601 in
     Primary Cutaneous Melanoma: Case Report"
     Front Oncol. 2020; 10: 1056.
     Published online 2020 Jul 10. doi: 10.3389/fonc.2020.01056
     PMCID: PMC7367153
     PMID: 32754440

40   Sarah Sammons, 1 Donita Brady, 2 Linda Vahdat, 3 and April KS
     Salama* 4
     "Copper suppression as cancer therapy: the rationale for copper
     chelating   agents in BRAF V600 mutated melanoma"
     Melanoma Manag. 2016 Sep; 3(3): 207–216.
     Published online 2016 Sep 2. doi: 10.2217/mmt-2015-0005
     PMCID: PMC6094647
     PMID: 30190890

41   Tam, P.B. "Tom Tam Bio" November 16, 2010 Tong Ren Station
     tongrenstation.com

42   Guidara, Juliette "5.4% - Beating the Odds of Cancer" September 23,
     2012

43   Tam, Tom "Healing Cancer With the Nervous System" Oriental Culture
     Institute 2012
     Pages 17-19 Biochemistry vs Bioelectricity

44   Tam, Tom "Healing Cancer With the Nervous System" Oriental Culture
     Institute 2012
     Pages 23-25 The Nervous System's Function

45   Tam, Tom "Healing Cancer With the Nervous System" Oriental Culture
     Institute 2012
     Pages 32-59 Meridians Are the Highways for Chi

46   Tam, Tom "Healing Cancer With the Nervous System" Oriental Culture
     Institute 2012
     Pages 146-48 Focus on the Diaphragm for Healing

47   Faruck L. Hakkim,1,6,* Hamid A. Bakshi,2,3,8,* Shabia Khan,3
Mohamad Nasef,2 Rabia Farzand,4 Smitha Sam,5 Luay Rashan,1
Mohammed S. Al-Baloshi,7 Sidgi Syed Anwar Abdo Hasson,7 Ali Al
Jabri,7 Paul A. McCarron,8 and Murtaza M. Tambuwala8
"Frankincense essential oil suppresses melanoma cancer through down
regulation of Bcl-2/Bax cascade signaling and ameliorates heptotoxicity
via phase I and II drug metabolizing enzymes" Oncotarget. 2019 May
28; 10(37): 3472–3490.
Published online 2019 May 28. doi: 10.18632/oncotarget.26930
PMCID: PMC6544398
PMID: 31191820

48   Bo Cao,1 Xi-Chuan Wei,1 Xiao-Rong Xu,1 Hai-Zhu Zhang,2 Chuan-
Hong Luo,1 Bi Feng,1 Run-Chun Xu,1 Sheng-Yu Zhao,1 Xiao-Juan Du,3
Li Han,1,* and Ding-Kun Zhang1,*
Atanas G. Atanasov, Academic Editor and Derek J. McPhee, Academic
Editor
"Seeing the Unseen of the Combination of Two Natural Resins,
Frankincense and Myrrh: Changes in Chemical Constituents and
Pharmacological Activities"
Molecules. 2019 Sep; 24(17): 3076.
Published online 2019 Aug 24. doi: 10.3390/molecules24173076
PMCID: PMC6749531
PMID: 31450584

49   Dr. Colin Champ, MD CSCS
www.dietdoctor.com-authors-drcolinchamp
colinchamp.com

50   Miriam Kalamian
Keto for Cancer - Dietary Therapies LLC
www.dietarytherapies.com

51   Maggie Jones
www.cancervme.com
Evidence-based nutrition and metabolic therapies

52   Dr. Judy Seeger ND
Detox and cleanse specialist
www.judyseegerdetox.com